A Jewish Mother's Guide to Professional Worry:

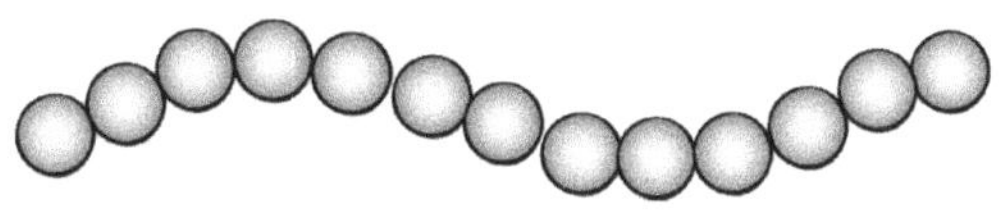

Worry Yourself to Good Health

as told to

Steve Malkin

Igloo Press, Tucson, Arizona
www.igloopress.net

ISBN 0-9787608-0-8

Cover design:	The Merry Wolf Studio, Tucson, Arizona (www.themerrywolf.net)
Cover painting:	Doug Weber, Tucson, Arizona
Text design:	The Merry Wolf Studio, Tucson, Arizona

Worry, worry, worry, worry, let it go.

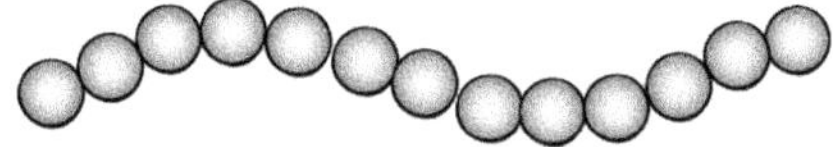

Introduction

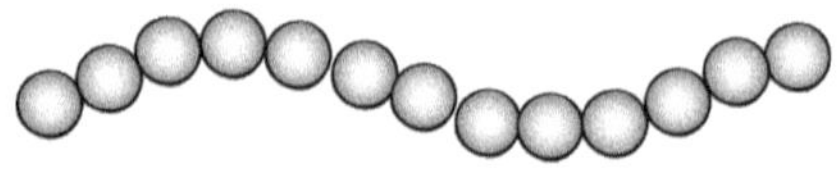

My mother Pearl is a professional worrier. She is an eighty two year old Jewish woman, who, when faced with all kinds of threats – divorces, cancer, children's illnesses, etc. – has pretty much emerged unscathed by the scoundrels and demons that haunt us all.

Her four children never really understood or respected her level of professional worry When we were growing up, we saw her worry all the time. Each of us unconsciously imitated her, *but without* the proper tools and techniques. I felt her pain, cried, threw tantrums, and went into fits of depression, believing this to be the right way to worry.

She would get us to worry with her, but we would always go too far.

It occurred to me that the children of the professional worrier have not been truly trained to worry their way to health. You know, like the cobbler's children have no shoes.

I realized worry was an art form which my mother had perfected over the years. By now, she was a true professional.

At eighty two, Pearl still plays tennis, rides horses, travels and takes care of her grandchildren (and half of the rest of the world).

Meanwhile, Pearl's children slowed down years ago, plagued by various illnesses ranging from bad backs to cancer.

I think our problems came from not appreciating her underlying perspective of how to worry in a healthy way.

My mother worries with concern, but without fear. She doesn't obsess. While my family went through all kinds of difficulties and upsets over the years, Pearl would hold it all together.

The idea for this book began when I spent my only vacation in four years at the John Wayne Cancer Clinic. The clinic is around the corner from Hollywood, in Santa Monica, California—the cancer clinic to the stars. My brother Marc had been diagnosed with melanoma, and our family gathered to spend time with him.

My mother had just arrived from the airport and was in the waiting room, talking to other cancer patients. Soon she was meeting with doctors in their offices, and hovering near the operating room. Pearl was down in the cafeteria, and outside in the street, talking to people about her son's condition.

I'm not sure, but at one point I could have sworn that she was talking to the huge lifelike memorial statue of the Duke himself. Yes, I think my mother was trying not only to get him to worry about my brother, but also to worry a little more in general.

The Duke was not the world's greatest worrier you know. He could have used some coaching from Pearl. "Hey, Pilgrim, what are we going to do about Marc's melanoma?"

As I watched my mother go into full scale professional worry mode, I also closely observed her ability to worry with detachment. Later, in the doctor's office, she encouraged another lady – Anna, to talk about her six operations, and her many returns to the clinic. Anna shared stories, about her life back in the Midwest, her children, her family, and how they were coping with her illness. She also told Pearl stories of her childhood, problems in her marriage before she became ill, and tales of various infidelities. You name it.

I could barely listen without great embarrassment, pain, sadness and debilitation. My mother, however, seemed to be glowing in rather a strange way. I was under the waiting room desk after hearing each of these stories, but Pearl was in her element. She was clearly supposed to be there.

After quite some time, Pearl involved Anna in listening to her worries about Marc's cancer, releasing Anna from dwelling on her own worries.

Before I knew it, while I hid under the coffee table as if in a high school air raid drill, my mother filled the entire waiting room, talking and worrying about Marc's condition. Pearl had somehow turned the Doctor's waiting room into a combination of gossip corner and cancer awareness workshop for her son.

As everyone continued crying and talking, Pearl once again amazed me. She zigzagged between nurse's stations, the Doctor's office, back out to the nurse's station, and back into the waiting room. *Pearl, who a few hours before had been carried into the hospital after she fainted in the street, was everywhere.*

She was making sure that, at least for that day, everyone in the John Wayne Cancer Clinic, and for that matter, in the immediate Santa Monica area, was at least thinking of, if not worrying about, her son's melanoma.

I realized that my mother was part of a lineage and tradition of women who learned to worry their way to health and long life. I decided to watch, learn, and take notes. Instead of the over-dominating, nagging mother I thought she was, Pearl was truly a survivor, a full-fledged professional worrier.

The problem all along was me. Over the years, I'd been debilitated by her worrying. I screamed, threw tantrums, ran away from home, become ill when she was sad – all in an attempt to do something about her multiple worries. I even developed an ulcer – something she herself has never had.

I tried to save her, to heal her; I rebelled; I was ashamed.

Then suddenly one day, I realized that this Lucille Ball of a mother actually had a method to her madness. *Worrying was her key to staying healthy and full of life.*

In the early years, I clearly did not understand the true nature of healthy worrying. I did not realize that, like a great Tibetan monk or Indian guru meditating on a Himalayan mountain top, my mother was doing her worry mantra.

Pearl was a master. She was okay. Her worry was okay. Her worry had purpose. *Her worry was intentional, instinctual, and methodical.* I watched. I learned. Now I know. I offer you some of the techniques and benefits of my mother's worrying, including her top ten worries and her ten commandments of the profession.

I even provide her resume, just to *kvell* a little.

I describe some of the pitfalls of ineffective worrying, discuss great worriers I have known, and even touch upon people who should have worried but didn't. I evaluate the different cultures of worrying, and, finally, tell how to worry yourself into a state of grace.

More importantly (and who could stop her?), I let Pearl do the talking.

As a reader, you might wonder what you should worry about. For starters, worry about not getting the full value of Pearl's teaching.

Being eighty-two and a Jewish mother gives me the right to be the subject of this book, since I have been a worrier most of my life.

Even as a girl, I worried. I worried if a boy would call me, worried if my folks would die, worried if I failed a test, worried if I was pregnant, and a million things more.

My mother Grace was a worrying-type person. She taught me well. Not that she taught me anything else – but she taught me how to worry.

Later, I worried if I was marrying the right man, if my children would be born healthy, and if they would grow up to be happy and successful.

I must say that this worrying did not hurt my health at all – in fact, in many ways, it got me through some of the most difficult periods of my life.

Many people say, "Don't worry," or "You worry too much." I say, "It's okay to worry." As a matter of fact, it's actually good to worry if you learn to do it like a professional. Like a good chicken soup, it takes just the right ingredients.

As in any other pursuit, profession or athletic achievement, worrying must be done diligently. Most people worry and don't realize that there is a right and wrong way. In this day and age, being a professional is the only way to achieve success and stay healthy. At eighty two, healthy as can be, I can actually say I am a professional worrier.

Even learning how to worry a little bit is better than no worry at all. It's like taking antibiotics or getting a shot to build immunity against measles or polio. Professional worry will help you deal with everyday problems as well as more serious problems when they come along. Everybody has troubles. Why not learn to deal with them in an effective way?

I have learned to worry professionally, and I have chosen to share with my son some of my long-secret tips and suggestions for healthy worrying. My son has chosen to share them with you.

If you follow some of these tips, you can worry and stay well without a therapist or a doctor, maybe even without high blood pressure, your whole life long. Naturally, if you don't follow these directions, everything will happen to you and I'll really worry about you then. So listen to your mother!

Listen To Your Mother

Steve's Story

When I was growing up, and my mother would launch into her worrying, I just didn't get it. I guess that most sons and daughters do not understand their mother's worrying either.

In the 60's many of us were told, "Don't worry, just let it go." What we should have been taught was how to worry effectively.

I realize now that Pearl was doing her job. I would do well at age fifty to observe, to learn, to watch, to pay attention, to, god forbid, "listen to my mother."

Many sons and daughters are so busy either putting down their parents and grandparents for worrying – or rebelling against them – that we have never really considered the value or learnable techniques for worrying.

We have become worry avoiders and worry

critics, without really ever seeing the actual beauty of pure professional worrying.

I used to worry about her worrying, and I wasn't the only one. Often when people see my mother worrying, they think she is plagued with doubt and lack of faith. Witnesses to her worry confuse healthy worry with a more obsessive and destructive kind.

Very often, those who lack faith themselves feel threatened and, in turn, misunderstand my mother. They don't know from the professional worrier.

The truth is, it is possible to worry in a healthy way, with doubt. Part of a Jewish mother's job is to worry loud and clear, like a rooster crowing at dawn. If my mother *doesn't* worry, then people should really think something is wrong and that she doesn't love them. Ergo: *I worry, therefore I am.*

Most people don't realize that while my mother is worrying to prove her love for us on the surface, deep down, she has a profound, abiding faith that everything will turn out fine.

Remember - it takes a lot of faith to doubt. It takes a lot of faith to worry as much as my mother does. It takes even more faith to listen to her worry.

If you lack faith, worry can seem very frightening and very negative. So keep the faith.

I used to think that sharing worries with others was like gossiping. Now I know: worry is not gossip. Worry has to be shared very carefully.

A professional like my mother shares her worries in a way that people can forget in about five minutes. Pearl's professional worry sharing relieves her, and enables the recipient to feel a little bit more aware than they were feeling before – especially if they share their worries with her. When you're done reading this book, feel free to do just that. Share.

Write to Pearl at Pearl Malkin, c/o C.O.D. Ranch, Post Office Box 241, Oracle, Arizona 85623. If she doesn't hear from you, she'll worry that you didn't like her book.

Chapter One

My Mother, My Guru

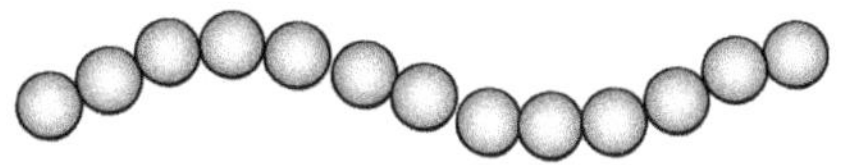

Pearl's Ten Commandments of Worry

One

Thou Shalt Eat Chocolate Ice Cream,

and chocolate in general. Medical studies have shown that it has a calming effect on the body.

Two

Thou Shalt Eat Chocolate Ice Cream in a Hot Bath.

Don't get too fancy about it. Massages, jacuzzis – forget 'em. Just a simple hot bath and a bowl full of ice cream will do - maybe a little whipped cream and nuts.

Three

Thou Shalt Worry with Love and Gratitude.

Always worry with love and love your worries. Remember that wherever your worries take you, spice them with love. Every worry presents a new opportunity to love.

Four

Thou Shalt Not Medicate.

Antidepressants and worry don't mix. Some people take pills in the face of upsetting situations. It is difficult to worry effectively when using too much medication. Sometimes, it is better not to worry at all until you are feeling a bit stronger. Wounded or medicated worriers can't seem to worry as well. Wounded worriers turn worry into an obsession. If you have to take medication for extreme situations, that's fine. When you are feeling better, start worrying.

Steady, daily worrying can sometimes do more good than antidepressants.

Five

Thou Shalt Exercise Your Worry.

All the time. Remember that healthy worry is like exercise. Done in the right proportions, it can strengthen you. Worry a little bit all the time. A little worry here; a little worry there. Even when things are okay, worry a little bit. Worry is like a muscle you must keep in shape. That way when you really need it, the worry muscle will be strong. Like workouts in the gym, never overdo it – or you can get hurt. Just exercise a healthy amount of worry all the time. If you stop worrying altogether when things have turned out okay, you might later get caught off-guard. Then you'll need to begin all over again. I just read of a study which demonstrated that optimists do no better, and sometimes fare worse than others, when faced with a depressing or upsetting situation. This is a consequence of expecting the best rather than worrying along the way. Worrying well is like preparing for the worst and being relieved when it's not so bad.

Six

Thou Shalt Not Treat Worry Like the Leper of Emotions.

Include worry as one of the gang – i.e., lump it along with good thoughts, hope, positivism, love, and prayer. Worry invariably leads to prayer and ultimately to gratitude.

Seven

Call Your Mother.

Reach for the phone. After a hot bath, go into Pearl's long-term routine. Follow Pearl's recipe. Wear plain loose fitting clothes, make regular phone calls, and visit witness worriers.

Eight

Call The Next Best Thing.

Get a priest or a rabbi to worry about you. Many priests, I have noticed, are too depressed to be able to worry. And most rabbis are so worried about losing their job that they can't worry about their congregates. Don't let them off the hook. Like with Job, God wants us to worry. He wants us to have a sense of awe.

Nine

Watch Slightly Sad Movies, and Occasional Talk Shows.

Even if you do this mainly to see how most talk show hosts don't like to worry. They either want to make everything okay, or bring things to a head to create a dramatic explosion of conflict. Fortunately, there are still some good old-time worriers.

Ten

Slouch.

When engaged in a serious worry crisis, never stand fully erect. Lean a bit. Slouch. Look like a *schlemiel*. Who cares? Why wait for Passover? Recline. Slow Down. Walk slowly so as to slow others down and to get their attention. In these high-tech, high-speed sound-bite days, worry can bring people to a more natural state; a more familiar time and place. Become a healthy worrier. Maybe someday you can become a professional worrier. Then, when it's all over, stand tall. Put on your make-up, wear your best clothes, and hit the world running. Everyone will say, "After all she's been through, look how great she looks."

Chapter Two

Pearls of Wisdom: Profile of a Professional Worrier

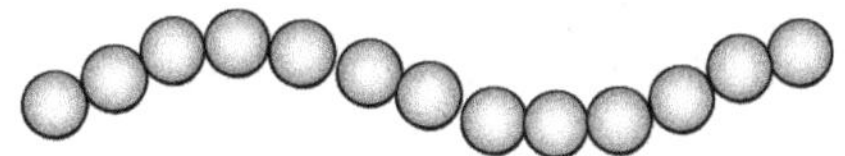

How Do You Tell a

Professional from an Amateur?

Conducting a Background Check.

Résumé of the Professional Worrier

Pearl Malkin
Resume of a Jewish Mother
2021 Ocean Parkway,
Brooklyn, NY

Objective: To speak the truth as I see it — to as many people as possible.

Education:
❍ Graduated top of her class from the College of Jewish Wartime American Princesses (JEWAP).
❍ Majored in Match-Making
❍ Minored in Chicken Roasting

Languages: Speaks her own special dialect of "Pearlese," beyond simple description, often indecipherable.

Work Experience:
❍ Professional Worrier and de facto author of the book, *The Jewish Mother's Guide to Professional Worry*, written by her son, Stephen Malkin.

❍ Mother of the author of the best-seller, *"How to Make Your Mother Worry Forever."* (Still unpublished — too worried to finish).

❍ Dog Placement Specialist.

❍ Renowned Psychic Reader.

❍ Dating, Marriage, & Family Counselor.

❍ Dried Flower Arranger (Fired for adding too many flowers to each arrangement).

❍ Public Relations Account Executive/ Murrieta Hot Springs Resort. Specialized in taking minerals and mud baths, complimentary massages, schmoozing at celebrity parties and playing tennis.

❍ Professional Beauty Consultant: Offered advice and makeovers whether wanted or not. (i.e., "You have such a pretty face — except for those eyebrows. Here, let me fix them for you!) Specialized in kidnap-makeovers of homeless women.

❍ Telecommunications Expert: Perfected the "marathon" phone conversation. Famous for never saying the word "good-bye."

❍ Wife, mother, and grandmother extraordinaire.

Strengths and Special Skills

❍ Uncanny appliance-dismantling ability. Capable of destroying any home appliance in seconds flat.

❍ Automobile Demolition Expert. Give me your tired, your poor, your four-wheelers.
❍ In-supermarket eating skills. Specializing in grapes, Doritos and Pecan Sandies.

❍ Laundry Specialist. Colored clothes bleached in no time flat. Turns whites a beautiful shade of pink.

❍ Retail Exchange Expert — Her motto: "Distract, Distract, Distract."

❍ Generous and loving beyond compare.

❍ Devoted mother, wife and best friend to thousands.

❍ Amazing sense of humor and zest for life.

References
❍ Eli the Butcher.

❍ Zack the Baker.

❍ Saul the Candlestick Maker.

❍ Her Kids. So, let them *kvell* a little.

Professional vs. Amateur: War of the Worriers

All worriers have crises. How the crises are handled separates the professionals from the amateurs. Here are some tips for when a crisis hits.

Professional worry isn't about making sense or explaining things away or about creating blame. It's just a way to create some relief when faced with a really threatening situation. It's also a nice way to make friends and meet people – especially if you are new in town.

Rule I: Get People To Worry With You.

(Pearl Remembers)

Once I was bleeding a lot. And I worried and worried that I needed an operation. I went to the doctor. Then I went to another. I got them to worry and worried some more.

Then I decided to call all my best friends and I

got them to worry, too. Then they got their friends to worry and they all worried so much that it made me worry less.

I talked to strangers at the grocery store, and got them to feel and worry. The more people you get to worry with you, the less you actually have to worry yourself. And of course, as it turns out, my bleeding stopped and I never did need to have that operation. Best of all, I made a lot of new friends. (A Hint from Your Mother: Write A Thank-You Note.) You have to thank all your fellow worriers and tell them that their prayers to God made you get cured. People would rather hear that it was their prayers that healed rather than their worrying.

Rule II: Never, Ever Wear Make-up When You Are In A Worry Crisis.

Grooming negates the fact that you are worrying. Make-up is a cover-up, and when you need to worry, the worst thing of all is to cover up your cares.

Also, never wear nice, good-looking, or stylish clothing when you are in a professional crisis. Always wear loose, old, dark clothing. It helps you get into the mood and creates more sympathy.

Remember: when you have to worry for real, wear loose things, preferably dark. Cotton is especially good, or velvet. Not rayon, and never polyester. You need natural material for real worrying. Put on your old *schmattes.*

Wear something wrinkled, and if possible something comforting and old. At the time you come out of the crisis, put on your best clothes and best make-up. You'll look stunning compared to before and everyone will say, "Look how great she looks after all she's been through."

Rule III: Eat Soft And Hot Foods.

Eat plenty of soup, preferably homemade – mushroom barley or chicken noodle. Soup and more soup. Drown yourself in soup. Borscht never hurt anyone either.

Go for sweet things. Snicker bars, Hershey bars, plenty of hot chocolate. Sunflower seeds with the shell on, pistachio nuts with the shell on. It can be relaxing to remove the shells while you worry. And besides, it gives you something to do while you are worrying. Be sure to vacuum the sunflower shells. Vacuuming is great for worrying. No potato chips – too fattening.

Eat Chinese food and share your worries with the waiters and the owners. For some reason they either like to listen or they feel it's part of their job as restaurant owners. Besides, often they send you a free order of egg rolls or something. Some of my best worrying has been done in Chinese restaurants. Eat, and enjoy like you're in heaven. As a matter of fact, I hope they have pistachio ice cream and Chinese food up there.

Rule IV: Listen To Music.

Put on sad music and moan a lot. It's okay to be a *kvetch* in the privacy of your own home. But most of all, say to yourself, if I worry a lot and do all these things, deep down in my heart I believe everything is going to be okay.

Fool yourself. Act worried, feel worried, and expect the worst, but truly know inside that God is watching over you and that things most of the time will be okay. The good news is that most things we worry about never come to pass.

The music you worry to must be slow, soft, sad and preferably classical. Not *The Flight of the Bumblebee*, or Rap music.

Even better, worry to no sound – silence is best of all. If you have to wait long for an outcome, older, funny television shows can make the worry bearable until the good or bad news comes.

Rule V: Expect The Worst.

It's easier and better for your health to think the worst. *Kinehora.* Worry every day a little bit, and when things turn out okay, you will be thrilled. Exhilarated.

However, if you are sure everything is going to be okay, and you don't worry, and things do not work out, you will get a bigger and longer-lasting shock that could make you ill.

It is better to be a worry person and get a happy surprise. When you get bad news, you are more prepared for it because you've already been worrying.

A little regular worry over a long time is also much easier on your body than worrying all at once, when you are shocked.

So worry a little bit every day and stay in shape. It's kind of like aerobics, a strong exercise program, or a meditation practice.

Rule VI. Don't Be A Showboat Worrier. One can abuse worrying just as one can abuse drugs and alcohol. One can over-worry, obsess or flaunt the ability to worry, just to be noticed. The worst thing you can do is to worry too much, to be a showboat worrier. That's arrogant, insincere, and more important, it doesn't get results.

Rule VII. Get Hard Cases to Worry With You. Ask a really depressed looking person about their problems. Get them to talk. As they go on, my mother shows her concern. The depressed person looks into her worried face and sees pure worry. The worry on my mother's face could have struck worry in the heart of Slobadahn Milosevich – even Sadaam Hussein.

To hell with Condeleeza Rice, The State Department should send Pearl Malkin to Iraq. One look at her and they'll all crack. It's contagious. My mother is the Bubonic Plague of worrying. She spreads it everywhere.

Rule VIII. Beware of Narcissistic Worrying. For a professional worrier, the key is never to get caught worrying about yourself excessively. We know that worry is ultimately for your own good. It should always be done as if you were worrying about someone else. If you are caught in narcissistic worry, or worry about yourself, immediately shift the focus.

Distract the observer. Immediately talk about a son or a daughter who had cancer. Tell a long worry horror story. Make one up. Do whatever you have to do to take the attention off of the fact that you were worrying about yourself.

Rule IX. Never Get Over-identified As A Worrier.

You don't want to be known as the town *kvetch.* The worry should be subtle and almost unnoticeable. It should grow on people. It should be almost like breathing. When I walk in a room of friends, they say "Oh no! Here comes Stephen the worrier!"

But when Pearl walks in the room, they say, "Oh isn't she a sweet caring person. Let's ask Pearl how she's doing." Bingo – the first question and she is off to teaching worry throughout the land – subversively, of course.

Never actually call worrying by name. It has a bad reputation. Better just to do it. If people know you are worrying, you are not worrying professionally. Worry needs to blend in with everyday life. It needs to be camouflaged. Excessive crying is not good in public for a worrier. It draws too much attention. Real worriers, like my mother, are really not sad. They get their sadness out, cry a little and then carry on. My mother is eighty-two and she plays tennis every day.

Rule X. Speak Your Worries.

Sometimes when Pearl is really worried, she'll talk to a telephone operator who is bored with her job. The right operator can be a perfect listener. Or better yet, a waiter or waitress. They are often touched by being trusted with such personal information. They become part of your honored "worry circle." Besides, they will listen a long time, expecting a good trip.

This was easier to do in the past, since nowadays people are in such a rush that they seldom have time to listen. But there are still pockets where simple and wonderful worriers can be found.

Rule XI. Adopt a Hypochondriac.

Even if their illnesses are made up, this form of worry can actually release a lot of tension and prepare people for worse medical situations in the future. Some professional worriers thank hypochondriacs for keeping the faith. I myself have even made up worry stories with close calls (but always a happy ending), and tell them at parties or in crowds.

Better yet, worry about a real illness. Go ahead, worry your *kishkas* out. You have Mom's permission. Adopt me. Like I said, I'm the world's worst hypochondriac.

(Steve Remembers)

When I was growing up, Pearl always told me to call so she wouldn't worry if I was going to be late. I would almost kill myself finding a telephone to call to say I would be late, and she would say, "Why are you calling so late? You woke us up!" I should have realized then that her worry was truly professional and not to be taken too seriously.

Throughout my life she continued to worry about my health, about my klutziness, about my allergies, my asthma, and the incurable bone disease I was supposed to die from when I was born. My mother took me to every doctor until she found one who said I wasn't going to die.

She worried herself to health in the process. As for me, I became an absolute hypochondriac. The good news is that I didn't die – not yet!

Rule XII. Go To The Doctor, But Know The Rules.

If you can't adopt a patient, adopt a doctor. As you know, my mother plays a lot of tennis. Mostly doubles. She has a hard time keeping a partner, because as each shot comes over the net, they can hear her screams of worry. Her partner doesn't realize she is just relieving the tension of the match. She is, in fact, a secret weapon for him. She rarely loses. She does, however, lose an occasional tennis partner who cannot stand her worrying on the court. It is, of course, their loss.

My mother is always telling me stories about other people's problems and illnesses. It used to annoy me, because I thought she was being negative. Now I realize she was releasing other people's worry she had taken on, and sharing the burden and responsibility. *Good for her.*

As a young boy, I once had a psychiatrist walk up to me at our summer home. Out of nowhere, he told me, "Your mother is crazy." She probably made him realize he should worry more with his patients. I think he couldn't take her worrying, which drove him crazy especially on the tennis court. She would usually worry in public, rather than alone with one person. This way she could spread the worry.

Psychiatrists, psychologists, physicians and lawyers are often paid to worry for you. They are often not good professional worriers, because they are usually insincere in their listening. After all, their ultimate goal is to make you stop worrying. We *need* to worry, and all they say is, "Don't worry!"

The problem is, of course, they don't know how to worry in a healthy way. Look at all the doctors and lawyers retiring early with ulcers and heart conditions. They really don't enjoy worrying with you. Therefore, you have to employ some special rules when worrying in hospitals.

Worrying at the Doctor's Office: Pearl's Survival Manual

I. Get the Doctor to know you and worry with you.

II. Get friendly with all the nurses. Get them to worry with you. Create a *doctor's office-family*. The family that worries together stays healthy together.

III. While you are in the doctor's office, call your friends to make sure they are still worrying. Make sure to speak loud enough for the doctor or at least a nurse to hear you.

IV. Worry in front of a Doctor as much as you can. Begin in the waiting room. Get everyone talking about your problem, so the Doctor comes out just to see what all the fuss is about. In my mother's case, she's caused hilarious laughter, just to get the nurses' attention. Make sure the nurses won't forget you. In time they will treat you like royalty - or a least like a relative.

V. Get the desk nurse involved and away from her computer. Ask her a question. Cry, tell an off-color joke, do whatever you have to do to get her away from her paperwork. When you finally do get to see the Doctor, your reputation should precede you. "So that's the famous Pearl Malkin!"

VI. Make the Doctor worry. If you are calm when you walk into the examining room, he won't want to help you. Get the Doctor to worry with you. My mother used to love her doctors, especially her gynecologist. Once, she had a party and invited all her doctors to her house. They all spent the evening talking about their most difficult, unusual patient: Pearl Malkin. Her doctors would never forget her, and they were part of our family. They would do anything, as well, for Pearl's family. BUT… there is the matter of these young, arrogant HMO doctors. When Pearl went to her first HMO, she was assigned a young doctor from the East Coast. After a few visits, he lost his composure and screamed at her, "Mrs. Malkin! I moved 3000 miles to get away from my mother, and now she is standing right in front of me! Please, I just can't take this." For the longest time, this doctor would not interact with the Medical Snake Charmer, Pearl

Malkin. My mother had met her match in the form of a HMO Doc. She would joke, worry, complain, confront, but mostly worry about the fact that she could not reach this young doctor. Finally there was nothing left to do but create a severe case of shingles to get his attention.

At first, the medical bean counter didn't seem to give a damn. Weeks went by with no results. Many phone calls to her children and many painful nights passed. The young doctor seemed indifferent. Each time she came to see him, she was in more pain.

One day, the doctor walked in and saw my mother crying in great pain. He finally started to worry about her. He said, "Mrs. Malkin, you are exactly like my mother." Then he broke down and started to cry. He became her good friend and he is still her favorite doctor and she is his favorite patient. Well, at least he sincerely worries about her.

VICTORY FOR PEARL! She won. Not only for the sake for her own health care, but in some way, she did more in this one moment to humanize the HMO system than Hillary Rodham Clinton ever dreamed. If each person worked on their HMO doctor like my mother has, getting them to worry a little bit more, we'd have a more compassionate healthcare system. I'm convinced of it.

How about a little worry, Doc?

When my brother was sick with cancer, Pearl would walk around without make-up, in her oldest clothes, just waiting for someone to ask her how she was or what was wrong. Even the perfectly groomed waiter of the elegant Italian restaurant we went to for lunch was recruited to worry. The restaurant soon became a chorus of worriers for her son's recovery.

Most of all, the real prize occurred when the Doctor would ask Mrs. Malkin, "Do you have any questions or concerns?" The poor doctor had no idea who he was talking to. We need doctors who worry like they did in the old days. We don't need ice-cold technocrats, or these new all-star know-it-alls. They give seminars. But they stopped really seeing patients. "Don't worry, there is an herb for this," they say.

"Don't worry, there's plenty of tree bark in the Amazon for this. Think positive, meditate. It's all in your mind. Read the right poem, find the perfect remedy, and you will be fine. If not, perhaps you've caused your own illness." Or – read my book and you will feel better. Wait a minute, that's what Pearl says. How about a little worry, Doc? Write fewer books, present fewer seminars, and start worrying about people again. I am seriously thinking about bringing my mother to one of Dr. Deepak Chopra's or Dr. Andrew Weil's seminars so she could start to work on them.

Pearl could ask a few questions, and get them to start worrying a little . . . to add that missing ingredient. Right now, they're probably just worrying about having to pay taxes on all the money they're making.

We don't need guru doctors. We need doctors who know how to worry. When an HMO Doc explains, with Latin prefixes, all the reasons to stop smoking, I hardly listen.
But if I look in his face, and he really looks worried, I say, "Doc, what's wrong?"

When I see my doctor worry, I really begin to listen. If I see a surgeon worry, I listen even more. And if I see a hospital administrator or an insurance rep worry, I run for a priest or a rabbi.

Pitfalls of the Professional Worrier

I. Beware of Despair.

Recently, I saw my mother get very upset about my financial situation. I am an expert at triggering my mother. I am the one person who can dismantle her professional worrying. And when I do so, her worrying can turn into despair. Beware of professional worriers who can slip into despair. It can happen to the best.

- Despair has no real focus.
- Despair is pure upset, with no secret pleasure in knowing that things will probably be okay.
- ·Despair has no discipline at all.
- You can't despair for very long.
- ·Despair becomes random and epidemic. It can turn into real illness. Despair can also cause the chicken-little syndrome; "The sky *really* is falling."

- It's hard to worry too long about very large catastrophes. They are too broad and too frantic. Healthy worry has a rhythm, and some comfort. No flailing or gnashing of teeth. Worry never says, "This is the end of the world."
- Don't worry about the end. Take comfort in the fact that there really is no end to worry.

II. Worry Is Not Depression.

Healthy worry can counteract depression. I have hardly ever seen my mother actually depressed. She can't afford it, she has a job to do. She is a professional worrier, like a golden retriever returning a bird or a stick.

Orthodox Jews move their body up and down when they pray, something called *davining*. My mother moves her mouth up and down instead, spreading the word in a proactive way. She's always on the go, actively worrying.

Healthy, passive worrying is possible, but only for the most advanced worriers. Healthy, passive worrying fits into the category of mystical worrying. And should only be limited to a select few worry gurus. For the most part, worrying must be active and practical.

III. Never Fail To Acknowledge Fellow Worriers.

If you see someone worrying in a healthy and professional manner, following all of Pearl's rules, then give a knowing nod, and cheer them on – subtly, of course. Acknowledge them; know that you are in the presence of a pro.

But don't spend too much time with them. It's like two angels meeting and going out for a beer. You each have work to do. You need to go out and worry with non-worriers.

Of course, as a professional, one or both of you may have shut down and stopped worrying or become caught up in worry atrophy. Like two great athletes working out together, it couldn't hurt to spend a little time worrying together just to get back on track. Then be on your way.

Remember, you were given a brain to worry, use it. You were born to worry, so do it right.

IV. Distinguish Good Worry From Bad Worry. One time a friend of mine who owed me $30,000 came up to me with the money to pay me back. At the time, I was being audited by the IRS. I was so worried about the audit that I told my friend to keep the money for a few weeks. The audit was over and by then my friend had gone bankrupt. I never did get the money. This was a good example of letting worry turn into fear and dysfunction. It's an example of worry gone bad. Never let worry stop you from moving forward and collecting the money.

During the Cuban missile crisis, I sat in front of the TV, certain that there was going to be a nuclear war. I stayed in the basement and didn't move for about ten days. Finally, my father came downstairs and asked me what I was worried about. I said we were all going to die.

He gave me a prayer to memorize about the difference between what can and cannot be changed, and the wisdom to distinguish between the two - or something like that. After two weeks, I finally got up and went to school. Again, I hadn't yet learned to worry.

Where was Pearl during all of this? Probably out playing tennis.

V. The Role of Historical Worry.

If you can't find anything else to worry about, remember your history. Consider a particular WWII battle, or the question of who killed JFK. Better yet, bring up something more private and personal in your past. Get into it as if it were the present.

Historical worrying is not as good as here and now worrying, but it is better than not worrying at all. Of course it's better to pick a historical worry that turned out okay. Bad endings can ruin a good worry. But if you look back in history, you'll see there's no end to worry. The art of worry is one of *knowing how*. Remember, always spread worry gently. Also, pick catchy phrases or worry mantras, like "God forbid, *kinahora*," a Yiddish expression that means "knock on wood." Worry well.

VI. Beware Of The Phantom Limb Syndrome. Remember your history, but don't dwell on the past worries. Amputees often feel pain in a limb that's no longer there. Similarly, the phantom limb worrier gets plugged into worries that are long gone. This can complicate worrying in the present, which is truly the only real kind of effective worrying. If you get caught up in a phantom limb worry, come back to the present. This is the biggest pitfall of them all – worrying about things that have nothing to do with the present situation. The only redeeming value is that at least, you are still worrying. But get a grip. Come back to the present! Remember – there's enough to worry about in the moment.

VII. Don't Lose Your Sense of Humor.

My mother never stops telling jokes. A great way to walk into a group of strangers is to get them laughing. Laughter has always been a great form of release. Much humor comes out of worry. Don't think worry and humor don't go together. They do.

VIII. Remember to Worry Long Distance.

If you can find one, a good phone booth is a great place for long distance worry. It's dark, crowded and public. A good pay phone worry at the right time can be worth its weight in gold. Like the Clark Kent of worry, you become "Super Worrier." As the coin drops into its slot, the adrenals start pumping.

Phone booth worrying is the next best thing to worrying in person. Cell phones are a little too easy and accessible. Email, too impersonal and detached, is also prone to worry surfing and lost worries.

An excellent worry phone opportunity is in the waiting room at the doctor's. Remember to speak loudly enough so everyone in the waiting room can hear what you are saying. This obviously kills two birds with one stone. You can speak directly to the person you are worrying with. You can also pick up a few additional vulnerable worry witnesses, who are anxiously sitting in the waiting room.

IX. Give Up the Illusion of Control.

The dangerous or unhealthy worrier (amateur)

is the worrier who thinks he or she is in control. This can result in ulcers, cancer, depression, boils, frogs, and other Old Testament maladies brought on when things turn out differently than you have willed them.

For example, a heart attack can occur from the shock of things turning out differently than you thought or willed they would.

Remember that you are a professional, but *you are never in control.* Better words for worry are "pray, beg, hope, cry for, make a promise to God, if things turn out okay."

Know that you can't keep all the promises that you make to God. But just do your best. He knows you made them as a worrier. However, a true professional will try to keep their promises. Don't make ridiculous ones. Often I have seen people make absurd promises, when they were worried – promises they could not possibly keep. This is very unprofessional and bad for future worries.

X. Don't be Demanding.

The worst kind of worrier is the demanding worrier, the one who says: "I demand that you heal my mother. I order you to heal my sister. I insist that you make this surgery come out all right."

Worrying is a more gentle process. It needs to be done with humility.

XI. High-Tech/Low Tech/No Tech.

The downside of computers is that novice worriers could begin to think that their problems are erasable from more than just their hard drive – and that there is no need to share their worries. This notion can discourage healthy worry, which is often repetitive, like some kind of prayer or meditation.

Ultimately, erasing your worry is a good end. The danger is that you will avoid the all-important process, skipping the means and the technique. The computer has great potential for increasing the number of fellow worriers, but it must be done with heart. Otherwise, only gossip and fear will be spread, with not enough compassionate feeling.

Computers have done a lot for worrying. I seem to see people worrying all day long about their down computer. This, at least, gets people started worrying.

Another difficulty with technology is, for the most part, worrying is slow, not hyperactive or made for sound bites, like most modern technology. There's no high-speed internet connection for worry.

The other challenge with technological worrying is that the worry must be sincere before it's ever easy or fast.

XII. Think Tabloids.

The news and other soap operas are too sensational, too violent for healthy worrying, and can create a certain numbing of one's worry sensibility. However, if you could get on a local television show and actually worry about something personal in a very human way, you could do a lot to further the cause of healthy worrying. Pearl has been on T.V. a number of times spreading healthy worry.

If you sprained your ankle yesterday and could get on a local television show, imagine! "Folks, I am really worried about my sprained ankle, please call in cures you may know." What an opportunity to get thousands to worry with you.

My mother reads the *National Enquirer*. I know it's because she thinks that magazines like these are spreading the worry, like she would do in the supermarket. I feel they go too far.

But what do I know, I'm not a professional. My mother reads this rag when she is in the bathtub or on the toilet, possibly to stimulate her worry. It may be that only real professional worriers can get value out of the *National Enquirer*, because they don't take it too seriously.

Amateurs like you and me should probably avoid tabloids or use them in small doses, like a shot of whisky or cortisone or a laxative. Tabloids should only be used in cases where you are absolutely having great difficulty worrying.

XIII. Don't Let Your Imagination Create Worry.

One day I drove into my ranch, which is in the Coronado National Forest in Oracle, Arizona. There's a good distance into the Arizona wilderness, nothing around for miles and miles. I saw that all the horses were now gone, along with the hay and the horse trailer.

The day before, I had left a rather harsh message on my wrangler's answering machine. I immediately imagined that he had packed up the horses and left the ranch for good. I worried all day, and imagined the worst.

Two days later, the wrangler showed up. It turned out he had taken the horses on a cattle drive. I went up to him and asked if everything was all right. He told me everything was fine.

It turned out I had made up the entire situation. I call this paranoid worrying. Pearl would say, "Don't use your imagination to conjure up worry. Don't make up worry. Try to worry about something real, that's a clear problem. There is no shortage of real things to worry about."

XIV. Avoid Needless Worry.

Most worries seem like needless worry. Especially if things turn out okay. Most people look upon worry over a situation which turns out to be nothing as wasted worrying. Why did I ever worry about that? Not to worry. There is a difference. Needless worry is the kind that creates panic and fear about some big abstract problem. Like Armageddon or a world war. Healthy worry is always more simple and specific.

Think of it more like practicing kung fu or some kind of training where you don't hurt your opponent or yourself. Needless worry can be somewhat healthy, as long as it's not obsessive or prone to create unnecessary fear or panic. But on the whole it is better to avoid this kind of worry. On the whole all worry in the end is needless, but it's the process that's important. It's the act of worrying that is important.

XV. Warriors vs. Worriers.

My mother says that on the whole, men are amateur worriers compared to women. They focus more on their careers, keeping a stiff upper lip. Men do not like being seen as worriers, and traditionally, are not good worriers. Historically, men go off to war, and women stay home to take care of the kids, worrying to keep the home safe. Thus, women developed a career of household worrying, and men became warriors. But in truth, the best worriers tend to make the best warriors. Think Colin Powell.

One of my hopes for this book is that after reading it, male leaders will listen to their mothers and become better worriers and more compassionate people. I hope men will learn some of the skills of worrying, and learn to worry more professionally. I hope that men will not be afraid of women who worry. Likewise, I hope that women will give men a chance to worry. Let men learn. It is possible. It just takes patience.

I also hope that women will bring their worries into the workplace and make corporations more compassionate. As more and more women join the workplace, I'm worried that this age-old skill of worry will get lost in the corporate wars.

Men who stay home can also take on some of the responsibility of worrying, which women have borne for so long.

They *Should* Have Worried

As I watched the very sad news about the untimely death of John F. Kennedy, Jr., his wife Carolyn and her sister Lauren, I come back to the role of worry. Remember, for starters, that Jackie Kennedy asked her son not to fly while she was alive. In deference to his mother's worry, he granted her wish.

Then, in the absence of the world-class women worriers in his family, Rose Kennedy and Jackie Kennedy, he felt he could fly to the wind, free at last to fly, and not to worry. Free from his mother's and grandmother's worries.

In reality, we are never free of the world-class worriers in our families. We would do well to listen to their wisdom, to learn from their worries. Even when they are gone.

If JFK, Jr. had worried about weather conditions, lack of emergency floats on the plane, visibility, etc., he might still be with us today.

Watching the news of this doomed flight on TV in a restaurant, I looked around and saw older and younger women watching the TV with me. Their eyes were glued to the TV, and some were crying. They all worried about JFK, Jr., and the Bessette family. With this new tragedy, these old worries about this family – which has become America's family – came to light again.

These women worried about the lives of the Kennedy children as if they were their *own* children. At this moment, they worried more about them than about their *own* lives. The Kennedy Clan once again validated the need for our nation to worry and to grieve together.

This tragedy tapped into a well of emotions. Strangers gathered at the New York City apartment of the couple to worry in public. The news media softened its stance. When we are united in our worries, we all become bigger than our individual selves in worry. But why wait for the grand tragedies? It's never too late to let a little worry into your life. A little bit of worry goes a long waythe wind, free at last to fly, and not to worry. Free from his mother's and grandmother's worries.

In reality, we are never free of the world-class worriers in our families. We would do well to listen to their wisdom, to learn from their worries. Even when they are gone.

If JFK, Jr. had worried about weather conditions, lack of emergency floats on the plane, visibility, etc., he might still be with us today.

Watching the news of this doomed flight on TV in a restaurant, I looked around and saw older and younger women watching the TV with me. Their eyes were glued to the TV, and some were crying. They all worried about JFK, Jr., and the Bessette family. With this new tragedy, these old worries about this family – which has become America's family – came to light again.

These women worried about the lives of the Kennedy children as if they were their *own* children. At this moment, they worried more about them than about their *own* lives. The Kennedy Clan once again validated the need for our nation to worry and to grieve together.

This tragedy tapped into a well of emotions. Strangers gathered at the New York City apartment of the couple to worry in public. The news media softened its stance.

When we are united in our worries, we all become bigger than our individual selves in worry. But why wait for the grand tragedies? It's never too late to let a little worry into your life. A little bit of worry goes a long way.

Chapter Three

A Little Worry Each Day

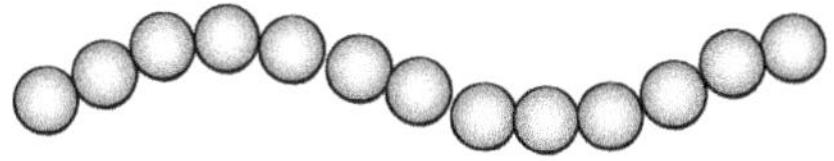

(Pearl Remembers)

My worrying days started at the age of thirteen. My mother told me I would get pregnant if a boy touched my breasts. Well, one day a boy dared to do that, and I worried. I worried myself into a fit.

It was then that I learned that certain kinds of worrying can make you ill. In fact, I did not get pregnant from a touched breast.

From that time on, I decided to learn how to be a professional worrier, rather than make myself sick. As a result, I have been healthy and happy since I was thirteen years old. It's a miracle-being Jewish and sensitive, and a real worrier, that I could stay so healthy.

And now at eighty-two, I'm disappointed if someone doesn't touch my breast! A real turnaround.

About 85-90% of the things I worried about when I was younger turned out to be okay. I found that I worried for nothing. Well, not really.

I always feel great after worrying a little each day. It's like building an immunity to disease, or working out in a gym.

The worrier slowly absorbs the worry and is prepared for the worst. The optimist, who is so proud of herself for always being so optimistic, gets the shock of her life when something goes wrong.

She hasn't built up her worry skills, and is unable to cope. In many cases the optimist falls apart, gets sick and cannot handle the stress. She cannot function in a crisis, and is, in fact, no use or help to others.

But if you worry a little each day, you are prepared for the bad news. You can cope without falling apart.

Hopefully, traumas will not happen too often in your life. I have been lucky and have had very few tragedies. Here are some tips I can share with you.

Pearl's Top Ten Worry Tips

I. Receive the impulse to worry. Welcome it. Do not view the worry impulse as the devil, negative energy, or darkness. Worry can be your friend, an angel telling you gently to pay attention.

Do not ignore your worries. Embrace them. If you ignore your worries, they will get louder and louder and turn into fear, guilt, anger, and obsession.

Healthy worry can prevent these emotions.

It is naturally humbling to worry.

Focus your energy on the problem.

Embrace worry when it comes into your life.

(Pearl Remembers)

All my life, I had had a fear of my husband leaving me. I was a young mother with three children when my husband, Irving, announced that he had fallen in love with another woman and was leaving the family.

I immediately got the children to worry. I took my oldest son, Stephen, to New Jersey to Lakewood Resort, and cried for two or three days, locked in the hotel room.

The children got so worried, that when their father came to take them to the amusement park on Sunday, Stephen made sure that none of the kids said a word to him. He was going to single-handedly get me and Irving back together, by hook or by crook.

I got Irving's mother so worried that she flew to Chicago to lecture Irving's new lover about the pain she was causing his family.

I got the rabbi to worry so much that he called Irving up and gave him a sermon about his responsibilities as a husband and father.

I got my father, who had Mafia connections, so worried that he got two of the "boys" to threaten Irving.

When I was all done, all I could do was put on my make-up, buy some new clothes, start dating, and get on with my life.

After three months of my carrying on with my life, Irving decided to come home. We had another child.

We proceeded to have twenty-five more years of marriage. When my husband was dying, he apologized for leaving, and thanked me for the years we spent together.

Having my husband leave me had been a lifelong fear. The fact that he went ahead and left me, and I worried intensely, in some ways ended this worry for me. I never really worried about this again.

Although it is rare, sometimes you can worry a particular fear away. Out of your life for good.

II. Look around to see if there are any ideal worry witnesses.

Be somewhat selective, because some of them will turn around and give their worries right back to you.

Question: *Won't people get mad if you are using them as a worry witness?*

Answer: *No, because you are stimulating their worry juices, and reminding them to exercise their worry muscles.*

At the Cancer Clinic, when my brother was sick, we were surrounded by seriously ill patients from all over the country. You could hear a pin drop in the waiting room. Tension filled the air.

Suddenly, bingo, enter Pearl. Lights, camera, action! She found another mother, Janie, sitting there almost numb, obviously an amateur worrier. Pearl got Janie to talk about her child and her child's numerous surgeries.

Before long, Pearl had Janie totally concerned and worried about my brother's melanoma. This might seem selfish on my mother's part, and in the past I would have thought so.

But with my new realization about my mother's uncanny abilities, I realized that she was getting this woman to worry about my brother so that Janie could detach and let go a bit about her own child. At the same time, Pearl could release some of her concerns and emotions around her son's condition. A fair worry trade.

Pearl was everywhere, involving as many people as possible in the process. When my brothers and sister and I entered the hospital, I watched how Pearl literally collapsed in our arms. We carried her into the hospital, thinking she would be out for a few days. Suddenly, like a revived Raggedy Ann doll, Pearl immediately snapped into action as soon as the Doctor came in. She left us all in the dust.

I thought we were going to have to take care of my Mother, and I was quite worried. Instead, she ended up not only taking care of my brother, but also his wife, his child, me, my sister, and anyone else within her reach.

In a matter of days, my mother was taking care of my brother's baby, doing laundry, talking to his young wife about the situation, dealing with me and my grief, patching up age-old family wounds and rivalries, and deciding who would drive with whom.

Later, at the end of the day, when we got to the parking lot, once again Pearl crumbled in a dramatic collapse. This time, I recognized that there was nothing to worry about. Or, I should say, this *was* something to worry about, but in my Mother's tradition, as a professional worrier. I learned that the greatest challenge is to worry professionally about somebody who is very close to you.

Sitting in a restaurant over lunch, I watched Pearl nurture a chicken Caesar salad, then send it back because it wasn't right. I watched her send back *my* dish because it wasn't hot enough, mainly in order to have more time to discuss my brother's cancer with the waiter. I watched her reorder my sister's lunch – just because she could.

Pearl was gathering worry witnesses wherever she went – widening her circle of worry. I knew I was truly in the presence of a master.

III. If there are no qualified witnesses to share your worries with, let yourself worry right to the point just before it becomes too painful. If it hurts too much, it's not professional or healthy worry. You want just enough worry to focus on the problem, and catch the attention of a passing angel. As a witness, even a family member will do.

Recently, my mother got into a head-on collision. Probably while worrying alone. As you will see, one of her cardinal rules is **always speak your worries** – never just think them. She demonstrated this *always speak* skill after her auto accident. An airbag had literally broken her jaw. The whole family worried: "What now? She can't talk, can't eat, can't worry."

We were really worried. She showed up to visit me with twenty notepads. And every two minutes, we had to look over to read Pearl's worry pad.

(Pearl Remembers)

A year ago, I had a head-on collision. I totaled my car (although it wasn't my fault), and the airbag broke my jaw. This qualified as a bona fide worry crisis, because, as a Jewish mother, I could not open my mouth.

I had to have my mouth wired shut and could not eat or talk for three months. I had to utilize all my skills to get through this one. I got the doctors to worry, I got my children to worry, and a large part of the community worried, too. I didn't speak, and as you know, one of the rules of worrying is to "Speak Your Worries."

What was I to do? I began to write messages to everything in proximity. No phone worry. No talk worry, which I had done all my life. I was forced to learn another way to worry – without using my mouth. I wrote my worries on pads of paper. After awhile, I could write very quickly. Besides, I found writing was a great way to get people's attention.

I moved in with my daughter, and in this silent

period, I realized I needed to pass some of my worry skills on to my daughter. As a disciple, she did quite well.

My main worry was that I was going to die of malnutrition, since I couldn't eat. I had spent most of my life dieting, and the good news – a result of this worry crisis – was that I lost forty pounds.

I almost forgot about my broken jaw. I was streamlined. I was quiet and svelte, and hardly recognized myself. Nine months have passed, my jaw has healed, and I am speaking again.

The only bad news is that I've gained back the forty pounds, but am back to dieting and playing tennis again.

Pearl returned to the Bay Area after visiting me for a while in Arizona. I was talking to her on the telephone, and she was telling me how badly her jaw hurt, how she couldn't eat, and because of the pain, she still couldn't talk comfortably. She was feeling great despair.

Totally concerned and upset about her condition, I even thought she might do something foolish like try to kill herself. While talking with her on the phone, I had tears in my eyes, my stomach hurt, and my mind was all over the place.

With fear in my voice, I said, "Mom, please don't do anything foolish. I'll fly there tomorrow to be with you!"

And she said in the most normal tone, "No, I can't do tomorrow, I have a tennis date at ten. Could we make it another time?"

Need I say more? She worried herself right on to the tennis court. Amazingly enough, a tennis ball hit her in the jaw. She was knocked to the ground. When she got up, after getting everyone with a radius of 300 yards to worry about her, she spoke. "My jaw feels great; the tennis ball knocked it into place!"

IV. Hold your worry and reach a comfortable level with it – one that you can sustain and perform daily.

Worry just enough to awaken your adrenaline, not to drown in it. After awhile, if you are not going too deep, you will begin to feel okay. Of course, never, never admit that it feels good. People need to think it is very difficult. In reality, all kinds of chemicals are being released in your body to make you feel okay when you worry correctly.

(Pearl Remembers)

When my husband Irving died, I started to date again. After being married for fifty years to the same man! So I went on my first blind date.

I answered an ad in the Personals column. I waited for my date to knock on the door. I felt like a young girl again.

When I looked through the door, my blind date

turned out to be a rather short Chinese man. I ran into the closet to hide. I hid and began to worry in the dark. After worrying for a little while, I came out of the closet. I felt great.

I went out on the date and had a really good time. Later on, I got very sad. I worried that he'd drop me because I was Jewish.

V. Bow down to worry.

Forget about positive thinking. Worry is externalized prayer. Worry on the outside, pray on the inside. Prayer is always deep in your heart. Worry is on the surface, appeasing the gremlins.

People always say, "Don't be so negative. Be positive." If you are positive deep inside and you are also positive on the outside, the gremlins will get hungry and look for trouble. Let them see you worrying. Pretend it's the end of the world. Be Chicken Little. Say, "The sky is falling," when in fact you know that the sky doesn't fall.

Feed the gremlins raw worry. They surely will come to feed. And, deep down inside, you will see the gremlins for what they are.

(Pearl Remembers)

When I found out that my thirty-three year old daughter Alexis had breast cancer, I needed to involve everyone I knew, and everyone I met, in the worry. I needed to use all of my worry theories of dressing, eating, and talking. I needed to put my medical worry techniques to practice.

This was an all-out worry crisis for two weeks, during which we were waiting to see whether the cancer had spread. We also waited to discover her prognosis.

When we found out Alexis' situation was serious, my husband and I picked up and moved to the Bay Area to be with her. The worry crisis turned into daily action and worry.

I realized I had to carry on a full life while worrying a little bit every day, and spending quality time with my daughter. The prognosis? The doctors gave my daughter a year to live.

Eleven years later, she is a beautiful, thriving, wonderful and healthy woman. Some of those doctors, on the other hand, are no longer with us.

VI. Don't be afraid. Worrying is not fear – although the two are often confused. Fear is internalized worry. Always keep the worrying external.

The worry is out there. Wear it like a Catholic worry bead. Hold it like it is a Guatamalen worry doll. *Never* let the worry in.

(Pearl Remembers)

One day I drove into New York City to pick up a childhood friend in front of the Plaza Hotel. I parked my car, walked into the hotel, and for some strange reason, the doorman asked me what I thought of President Lyndon Johnson.

I told him how sad I was about President Kennedy and how I wished that President Johnson had been shot instead of Kennedy.

I couldn't find my friend Phyllis, so I left the hotel, got back in my car, and started circling the block of the Plaza Hotel.

Suddenly, I heard sirens. Police cars came out of nowhere. I immediately began to worry that someone was in trouble. I came to realize that four police cars surrounded my vehicle and were signaling for me to pull over.

They told me to get out of the car and put my hands in the air, and I did so. They began searching me and my car.

I compressed a decade of worry into twenty

minutes.

When they opened my trunk and found my son's toy machine gun, I thought, "This is the end." I began to cry. I told the two FBI agents that I was just a housewife and a mother. I said that this was my son's toy machine gun, and to please leave me alone.

It turned out that President Johnson was attending a luncheon at the Plaza Hotel that day, and the doorman had reported me as a "suspicious character."

I worried so much in such a short time that even the FBI decided to let me go. They told me to leave the area and go home. Relieved, I parked a block or two away, had a Snicker's bar and a knish, and walked back to the Plaza to meet my friend. My worry was over.

I did learn that once in awhile, it's better to keep your mouth shut – even if you're a professional worrier. I met my friend Phyllis, we had a lovely lunch at the Carnegie Deli, President Johnson survived my assassination attempt, and I went on to have a lovely day.

VII. Remember. Worry and pain are not the same thing.

Healthy worry should reduce or eliminate pain. If you do master healthy worry well enough, you can even reduce the pain of others.

There is nothing worse, when you are facing a threatening situation, than for some *schmendrick* to tell you not to worry, to be positive.

Healthy worry *is* positive. For the novice, healthy worry at first will not feel comfortable. *Be with* the discomfort until you get comfortable.

(Pearl Remembers)

I was worried because my oldest son Stephen was the only one of my children who had not gotten married. On the occasion of his fiftieth birthday party, I read a poem voicing this concern. At the end of the poem, one by one, I singled out seven women in the audience who I thought would be potential mates for my son.

I looked over at one and said, "What about you, Debbie?" I pointed to another, "Don't hide in the corner, Pat." Then I looked at one more, "How about you, Susan?"

My son almost died of embarrassment.

However, over the next few months, he did date many of those seven women. He's still not married. But at fifty-two, he has achieved a real understanding of professional worry, and he is no longer afraid of a woman's worries.

I hereby extend an invitation to any single women. He's still available. Go visit him at the COD Guest Ranch in Oracle, Arizona.

VIII. Healthy worry, practiced correctly each day, actually prevents illness.

Healthy worry is a form of humility – an acknowledgement of how vulnerable we are. If you were a tiny mouse in a stampede of wild elephants, wouldn't it be natural to worry?

We are all pebbles of sand in the face of the universe. A little worry is natural.

Healthy worry is really the opposite of what happens on today's talk shows. Even soap operas are no longer good worry helpers, since they are less about worry and more about action and violence. Others just tell you to think positive thoughts.

(Steve Remembers)

In the old days, there was a show with Jack Bailey, called "Queen For A Day." Remember that? A lady with all kinds of problems would appear on the show and share all of her sadness and worries with the world. The worry continued for most of the show - twenty out of thirty minutes.

At the very end, with tears in our eyes, while we were worrying with each contestant, Jack Bailey stepped in and said, "You are now Queen For A Day." He gave the winner all kinds of flowers and gifts.

I was brought up in the fifties watching "Queen For A Day" religiously with my mother. We would cry a little bit with each other daily.

Little did I know then that I was being trained to carry on my mother's lineage. Now I realize what really helped the lady on "Queen For A Day" was not the gifts, the money, or Jack Bailey solving all of her problems.

Like a TV aerobics class, "Queen For A Day" trained people to worry in a relatively feel-good way. We knew things would probably work out for the sad lady. The act of worrying was like eating a Thanksgiving turkey, full of L-tryptophan, making everyone feel better, and preparing all of us for things to come.

Likewise, the old soap operas were more about worrying, with long double takes and extreme close-ups of people worrying.

Currently, the soaps have too much action, violence, rage, and sex. The daily dramas are action soaps serving up too much speed and attention deficit disorder instead of being good worry trainers. Worry should always be done slowly.

The same with today's movies. Most are action-obsessed, and do not value good old-fashioned worry. Whatever happened to movies with long, tear-ridden death scenes? Those were the only movies I ever watched.

IX. Worry about death.

I didn't realize then that I was learning how to worry about death. It is not always time for action. Healthy worry can lead to patience. Worry is a form of patience because you worry while you're waiting. Worry slows you down, so that you can think about prayer and patience. Worry about death will help you face it, and death may not be as fearful as you think. Never internalize this form of worry.

(Pearl Remembers)

When my husband was diagnosed with cancer, with three months to live, I was terrified. I worried and worried.

I was afraid of him being gone. I worried about having the strength to take care of him each day. I worried about how I would go on with my own life. I worried and worried, and got lots of help from lots of people.

As it turned out, we spent three of our closest months ever – talking, sharing, laughing, crying and communicating together.

Irving passed like royalty. The whole family gathered, and we spent an incredible time together.

Even the rabbi visited, and gave my son a bar mitzvah at my husband's deathbed. (Irving had always been upset that our youngest son Marc had never had a bar mitzvah.)

I learned that I did not have to worry about Irving, that he would be fine, and he is now in heaven. I also learned that I would survive just fine, as I am doing to this day.

I learned that I am a lot stronger and more resourceful than I thought.

X. Respect your worry.

Worry is the unacknowledged middle child, the Rodney Dangerfield of emotions. Worry gets no respect. Sure – prayer, patience, compassion; everybody loves them.

But when things really get down and dirty, who shows up right away, almost like a reflex, to save the day and prepare us to get through things? Worry. Don't take worry too seriously or it will turn into pain and illness. When you get an impulse to worry, embrace it. It's natural.

Don't dwell on it. Let worry in the door; make it your friend. Good old worry saves the day, and makes room for the other emotions. Answer the door when worry comes knocking.

(Pearl Remembers)

When I was thirty, I took the kids to a concert in Brooklyn, and I met a 21-year-old refugee from Hungary. Somewhere between Fats Domino, Jerry Lee Lewis and Buddy Holly, I began to talk to the refugee and listen to his stories about the Hungarian Revolution.

Before I knew it, he was in the car, driving back with us to Long Island. Andy moved into our attic apartment. The neighbors talked. My husband didn't know what to think.

The refugee, Andy, fell in love with me. He wouldn't leave. I worried about my reputation in the neighborhood. I worried about my marriage, and what would happen to Andy if we asked him to leave. I worried about what my children thought too.

Finally, I decided to help him find a job and an apartment, and help him get on his feet. He stole our radio and a few other things. We never heard from him again.

I learned to worry about refugees. I also learned that in the future, I don't have to bring them home with me.

Chapter Four

Village Worriers

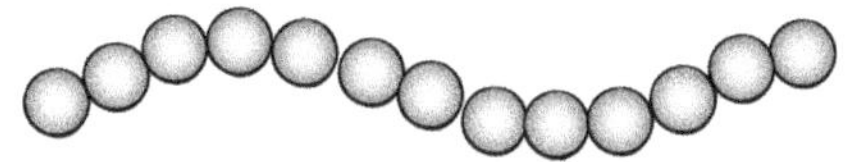

My Ancestors: Great Worriers I Have Known

My family is a bunch of *schtokers.* I'll start with my Grandma Maya, my father's mother. My Grandma Maya, at eighty-five years old, was truly a professional worrier. A survivor of Russian pogroms, she lived through the Russian Civil War, walked out of Russia just before Stalin took over, lived through the Great Depression, World War II, the Holocaust and the Korean and Vietnam Wars.

One day I saw her watching news clips of the Vietnam War in her living room. The war might as well have been in her living room on the sofa. No wonder she covered all her furniture with plastic. She was worrying about every step each soldier took, each shot she heard. At eighty-five years old, Maya, a survivor of all the above, was truly a professional worrier.

Growing up in the middle of two professional worriers was not easy. Each would criticize the other's style of worrying.

Maya felt things relatively deeply. Pearl seemed flightier and more shallow. I often struggled and tried to take sides. I did not realize that the fighting was merely about technique. Whose technique was a healthier way of worrying and more professional? Now I realize they had two different techniques of worrying. I also learned that it was hard for two or more professional worriers to live under the same roof.

Each knew what the other was doing. Of course, my mother had not lived through what my grandmother had, and therefore had developed a different style of worrying. Although each was different, they were both professional worriers. It was a clear conflict between Dostoevsky and Woody Allen.

Along with Maya and Pearl, were my aunts, Clara and Olga. None could agree on the correct technique. All of these women lived to a ripe old age. Their male counterparts, however, all died relatively young. The men in their houses would always say, "Don't worry!"

My grandfather, Maya's husband, died from a mistake the doctors made during a routine hernia operation. He should have worried a little bit about the operation - or even ear lice.

"Is this too heavy to lift?" A little bit of

worrying could have extended his life a long time.

I have seen my mother actually stop surgical procedures by running into the operating room and saying, "Wait a minute, are you certain everything is okay?"

Irving Malkin survived the Russian Revolution, the Russian Civil War, the Depression and the front lines of World War II. He once told me that after surviving World War II, it took a lot to get him worried. Nothing seemed as bad. So why worry.

My father would also say worry about that which can and should be changed, but accept that which cannot, and pray for the ability to tell the difference between the two. He seemed like the great non-worrier, with a gift for laughter and living life. A true *bon vivant*.

Later in life, when my father became ill, we realized that a little worry wouldn't have hurt him a bit, and that a stiff upper lip is not always the best way to survive. Broaden the worry. Share it with your family. Share it with the World.

(Pearl Remembers)

My husband Irving was lost in battle in Belgium during World War II, and declared "missing in action" for three months. I worried every day. Was he alive or not? I moved in with my mother and father, and spent every day with Irving's mother.

We all joined forces in an unlikely alliance, which only such a tragedy could create.

The mailman was our main worry witness, the target of our worries. Every day, we would ask him where the letter was.

I formed a team with Irving's mother, Maya, and though we had our differences, we pooled resources and worried together. The sheer force of two world-class worriers helped us each to survive the tragedy.

I worked as a gray lady and nurse for wounded GIs. Maya looked at each soldier to see if he was her son. After weeks of worrying, I realized it was my job to make the wounded soldiers laugh.

In the end, Irving was found alive and well in Belgium. The war ended. He came home and we began to make a life together.

The Village Worrier

During a period when there was a storm in Galveston, Texas, where I lived, my mother, living in California, wandered around a supermarket, telling everyone in the store about the storm, eating grapes as she went.

People gathered around the meat counter. Pearl told a joke, usually off-color, making everybody laugh, and then she called over the manager.

This enabled her to grab a few free grapes while they were laughing – maybe even a peach as the manager started laughing too. Then the flirting started.

Pearl meandered up to the counter to pay, engaging everyone in her conversation. The line slowed to a halt.

Remember Pearl's advice? Don't let anyone speed you up, especially when you are worrying.

Finally, someone behind her in line said, "Could you please hurry up and pay the cashier?"

Hurry up? Not a chance. Impossible. There's a whole story to tell the checkout lady, involving countless other people waiting in line. Maybe Pearl will even call in the manager, ostensibly to complain about something, but in fact, to involve him in the worry process.

The manager approaches. "Mrs. Malkin, is something wrong? You seem upset," he says. A perfect cue.

Pearl: "Oh my son is caught in a hurricane today, and I just don't know what is going to happen to him."

Person in Line: "Mrs. Malkin, I have a niece in Galveston. She says the news makes it worse than it really is."

Another Person in Line: "Don't listen to them. These news people don't know what they are talking about. Besides, my son is living in Bosnia now, and he is really in trouble." (Notice the worry escalation here.)

Manager: "Well, I heard things were getting better there now... But I certainly hope that your son is alright."

Pearl: "But he fixes houses for others, and he has a bad back. He never takes care of his back, and he works so hard." (Notice how she has compounded the issue, bringing in as many problems as she can in a short amount of time, and trying to fully engage the manager. For a moment, she stopped the world. A real pro!)

Pearl's grocery story worrying created a sense of community that did not exist there before. People continued to talk in line for quite a while.

Finally, a sound came from the back of the line. "Hey, could I please pay for the groceries and get the hell out of here?" At that point, the manager snapped out of his trance and came back to the present. He asked Pearl what she called him over to complain about in the first place.

"Oh, I can't remember," Pearl said as she swallowed a few more grapes she had been holding in the palm of her hand. The manager gave her a little hug.

People looked at each other as they stood in the line, which started moving again. The pace picked up and things returned to normal. But Hurricane Pearl did slow things up just enough with her worry to get people to talk to each other, and to care a little bit about each another. And hey, not to mention, she devoured a quarter of a pound of free grapes.

The Grapes of Wrath

(Pearl Remembers)

I just want everyone to know, that while I have certainly nibbled on my share of free grapes while wandering in the grocery store in search of fellow worriers, I am not a ganif.

I have worried about a touch of kleptomania in the past, but my worries brought things pretty much under control, and I limited my activities to grapes. It's been all about grapes. Anyway, that evening my son Stephen was telling you about before? Well, I prepared for New Year's Eve by wandering in a store in Marin County, California, a much fancier and lonelier village than Brooklyn, New York. I was grazing on my usual amount of free grapes when I was abruptly tapped on the shoulder by the store security guard who asked me to please "step to the back of the store."

Of course, I immediately began to worry. "Pearl," he said, "You're a very good customer and we don't want to prosecute, but our automatic eye camera photographed you stealing grapes. The store rules force me to report this incident. After the weekend, on Monday, we will let you know whether or not we are pressing charges."

Press charges! I couldn't believe my ears. The nerve, after thirty years of free grapes, I was apprehended like a common shoplifter. Didn't they know who they were dealing with? I am the village worrier; certainly entitled to a few handfuls of grapes. They made me fill out some forms (admissions of guilt), and sent me on my way.

Needless to say, I was worried beyond belief. This was an unusual kind of worry, because I was too humiliated to tell anyone I knew, except my family. I would have to call this a rare case of private worry.

I began to imagine myself on the Six O'clock News, in the National Enquirer: "Jewish Mother Apprehended in Marin on a Wild Grape-Eating Binge."

I spent my New Year's Eve preparing myself for the worst. On Monday, I was to begin my jail sentence. I called my son Stephen and told him I was arrested and going to jail. I made him promise not to tell anyone. This, of course, caused him to cancel all plans for New Year's Eve and go to bed worried about how he was going to get his mother out of jail.

On Monday, I went to see the Head of Security for this supermarket chain and their attorney. I finally had him feeling terrible and apologizing for what he had done.

They instructed me to either serve three days in jail or pay a three hundred dollar fine. I paid the fine and spent the first day of the New Year a free worrier, back on the streets.

Imagine! They should be paying me, the Village

Worrier, for spreading worry and helping people share their worst concerns. Instead, I have to pay them. Boy, times sure have changed. This would never have happened in Brooklyn.

Happy New Year and zei gesund.

Chapter Five

The World is Your Mishpacha

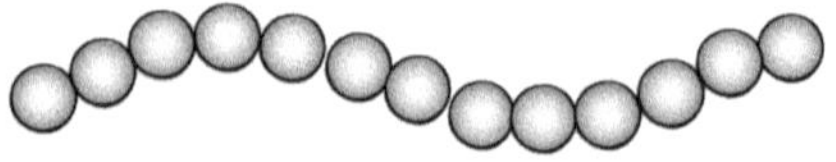

In a time when people are so concerned with borders, boundries and having their own space, Pearl Malkin wages an unending battle of butting into everyone's business and talking about everyone's problems. The world is her *mishpacha,* her family. Last month, while eating at a truly Manhattan restaurant, she and her daughter Alexis overheard a couple arguing at a nearby table. Pearl couldn't help but get involved.

When Pearl heard the wife complain to her husband about his behavior, Pearl leaned towards the next table and blurted out, "You know, you're lucky you have such a handsome man for a husband." At first, the perfectly-coiffed and well-dressed woman was shocked by my mother's interruption, since they had imagined they were all alone in a fancy restaurant.

Little did she know she was sitting next to a world-class village worrier. In a short time, the four of them were sitting at the same table, talking about marriage, relationships and each of their problems.

Pearl shared her own history with the woman. Pearl told her about the time when her husband left her, and described the trials and tribulations. She also shared the successful repair of her marriage.

After about an hour and a half of lunch and

marriage therapy, the couple thanked my mother and sister and offered to pay for their lunch. Pearl, of course, refused, because real Professional Worriers don't charge for services.

To some, it may appear that Pearl is violating another's privacy. What she is really doing is trying to make everyone realize that we all live in the same village, that we are all connected, and in many ways, obligated to care for each other and to share our worries with each other.

Worrying is one way to bring people together. I have watched my mother in restaurants, shopping malls, supermarkets, doctor's offices, and circus tents for my entire life. For many years, I was angry or embarrassed by her behavior. I finally realized that what Pearl is really saying is, "A village that worries together, stays together." My mother may have left the *shtetl*, but the shtetl has never left Pearl.

Council of Grandmothers

In the process of restoring an extremely run-down cattle ranch in the Arizona wilderness, I thought I was living out my male cowboy fantasies, formed as a result of watching too many "Lone Ranger" TV shows when I was a kid in Brooklyn. I think this is probably what got me to Arizona in the first place.

I thought I had created the perfect hideout next to Cochise's stronghold. The hideout where the Lone Ranger and Tonto hung out. The perfect hideout from my mother, my grandmother, my four aunts, the Long Island culture, and all it represented. I thought that I could become a real man in my desert hideout. Free at last, free at last.

Ironically, as the ranch became ready for guests and open for retreats, one of the first groups to discover my hideout was a group called "The Council of the Grandmothers." The "Council" was a large network of over two hundred mothers and grandmothers who gather every year to worry about all the problems of the planet.

The group practiced something called a "Spirit Circle," which was a gathering of approximately seventy women, ages fifty-five to ninety. They actually created what I would call a "worry circle," and proceeded to spend six days professionally worrying about the problems of the world.

Here I was in the middle of nowhere, surrounded by my mother times sixty. Like I really thought I could get away.

This reminds me of the story of the revered Tibetan guru holding court high in the Himalayan mountains, and the woman pilgrim who braved days and days of trekking in heavy wind and cold temperatures with scant food and water, to reach the summit.

The guru, who rarely granted pilgrims an audience, heard of her brave ascent. She took her place in the long line of other pilgrims who waited for words of wisdom from the great master. One asked about the nature of enlightenment. Another asked how to transcend pain and suffering. Still another wanted to be his disciple and yearned to be taught how to live a true ascetic's life.

Finally, the guru called this woman to come forth and asked her what he could do for her. The woman responded, "Sheldon, please come home already!"

Sons or daughters out there, listen. If you think you are going to run away from your mother's worrying, you've got another thing coming. Better to embrace it. It is your path to enlightenment!

Global Worrying

From India to New York, worrying is a global phenomenon. Here are some of its worldly manifestations.

Meher Baba, the revered Indian mystic said, "Don't Worry, Be Happy." Pearl Malkin, the eighty two year old Jewish mother from Brooklyn says, "Worry. Be Happy."

Worry Around the World

Jews: Excellent worriers. Sometimes take on too much baggage. Sometimes get attached to their cultural circumstances or their story, i.e. the Holocaust. Also sometimes take their worries too much to heart. Think they invented worry. Overall, excellent worriers – some of the world's best. Very good at consistent, steady worrying. But they need lessons to worry, worry, and worry, and then let it go.

Chinese: Very good worriers. Not good at

sharing worry with others. Can seem cold. Are actually very good worriers, tremendous discipline. Especially Chinese Christians. More so Chinese restaurant owners and waiters, who are among the world's best.

Christians: Super worriers. Sometimes faith can get in the way of worry, i.e., if you worry, you have no faith. Prone to martyrdom, which is the opposite of worry. Protestants tend to hide their worry as if everything is just fine, thank you. They might worry more to shake it up a little.

Tibetan Buddhists: Invented worry, i.e., worry beads. Sometimes too detached. Can become too automatic. Let it go too soon. Remember, *worry first* and then let it go. Some meditate instead of worrying.

American Buddhists: Sometimes let it go

before they worry. Many turned to Buddhism to get away from Catholicism and Judaism. Ran away from worrying and Jewish and Catholic grandmothers. Hoped in Buddhism to escape worry. Buddhists say you cannot escape from suffering. Pearl would say the same about worry. I would say the same about escaping from Pearl's worry.

Italians: Good worriers. Balance Catholic severity with a zest for life. Sometimes, because they live so close to the Pope, their worrying can be an imitation. They look good in black, which is an excellent color for worrying, and the women are not afraid to cry out loud. This ranks them very high on the worry scale.

Russians: In the past, Russians were good worriers. Communism discouraged it, but still there was plenty of private worry. Russians sometimes confuse worry with pain and suffering – look at the epic dramas they've written! Worry can lead to an excess of vodka or genuine release. Although they worry too deeply, there is great potential in the Russian worrier, especially the Russian Jewish worrier.

Spanish: They have a good base with Catholicism, and a good reminder in the Inquisition. However, modern Spain is very prone to fulltime partying since Franco. No time to worry. A reaction to oppression. Can confuse worry with repression. Great use of black lace. Complicated crosses and crucifixes. Huge intimidating churches. If they could only stop partying, the Spanish people could make great worriers.

India: Tend to worry all the time, which is both good and bad. Often worrying about becoming enlightened. Pearl says, "Best to worry about small things, and real human problems." Worrying about enlightenment can actually reverse healthy worrying. Enlightenment can overshadow worry and is not for everyone. Worry is for everyone.

British: They just don't worry. They conscript the Irish to do it for them.

French: Worry is *déclassé. Vin* and *fromage* are much more satisfying, *n'est pas?*

American Indians: Build the casino now. Worry later.

Jewish Indians: Forget about 'em, they're off the chart!

Japanese: They look like they're not worrying on the outside. So what's with the hara-kiri?

Hassidic Jews: They worry their way to miracles.

Irish: See "They Should Have Worried," page 66.

Rabbi's Resolve

In the Orthodox Hassidic tradition of Judaism, there is a technique for resolving questions about the Torah. Two rabbis sit across from each other at a table and argue, discuss and worry about each particular question in the Torah. They look at the question from every conceivable angle. The exchange goes on for days and days. Finally, at one point, one rabbi looks at the other rabbi, and they simultaneously shake their heads in agreement. At this point, and for this moment, a state of grace exists and the issue is resolved.

The Miracle in Oracle

One day I got a phone call from a group of Hassidic Jews from Crown Heights, Brooklyn, who had discovered my ranch via the Yellow Pages. They were preparing to host sixty Hassidic women from a girl's camp, the daughters of Hassidic Rabbis from remote villages around the world. The hosts had lost their original location. The girls were showing up in four days. Everyone needed a miracle.

I let 70 orthodox girls and 5 rabbis use my ranch. This in itself was considered a miracle in Crown Heights. A Jew in Oracle? The Hassidim have a habit of waiting to the last minute and then calling it "a miracle."

Just before they were to arrive, a building we had brought onto the property for them got stuck on a hump in the mud and was blocking the road, making access to the ranch impossible.

We tried everything to move the building—

digging, pushing, pulling. We even flagged down a crane which, miraculously, we saw in the area. No movement.

Still stuck. It began to pour rain. Out of nowhere, my mother showed up in a large travel trailer, with her new gentlemen friend, John – whom I'd never met. She started worrying instantly, and got John to also worry.

John turned out to be a nuclear physicist who was raised on a farm. He remembered how to hotwire machinery. Suddenly, I looked over at a part of the ranch where there was a pile of rubble and saw John rummaging through the junk, unearthing a broken-down backhoe.

He proceeded to hotwire the machine and drove it toward the stuck building. He lifted the building over the hump and pushed it out of the road, just as the busload of Hassidic daughters arrived.

What in the world was Pearl doing there?

Where did she come from?

When the Head Rabbi — who was the founder of the Hassidic Girl's Camp — arrived, Pearl ran up to him. "Hello Mendel," she said, and gave him a giant hug, which is forbidden in the Hassidic tradition. Although these rabbis had found us in the Yellow Pages, it turned out that this rabbi, Rabbi Mendel, was the same rabbi who had *Bar Mitzvah'd* my brother at my father's deathbed and presided at my father's funeral.

When the Hassidim heard this coincidence, they immediately called it a "miracle." All of Crown Heights, Brooklyn sang and danced. To this day, they still speak of the great "Miracle in Oracle."

The rain continued, everyone settled in safely, and when we looked up, Pearl was gone. She was worried about what Rabbi Mendel would think of her, sleeping in the trailer with a man she wasn't married to. I still have no idea what Pearl and her boyfriend were doing there, but everything worked out for the best.

As for the Hassidic Girls, they come to the ranch every year, and often ask, "Where's Grandma Pearl?"

Chapter Six

Worry Yourself to a State of Grace

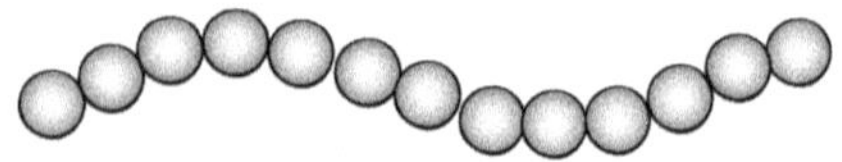

The Zen of Worrying

When I watch my mother worry, there is no illusion about some great profundity saving the world, or any great achievement. In fact, she is not very good about worrying about those kinds of things. She is simply worrying about her daughter, her son, her operation, the neighbor . . . and she knows that the outcome is not entirely in her hands.

However, her one little bit of worry could be the one thing that sways the outcome in a difficult situation. Everyone must do their part to get through a crisis. Kind of like: *It takes a village* to get through oral surgery.

When I was growing up, I was often near my mother's side as she worried, and even more so when she worried about me. I never realized how much of her worrying was to relieve her own discomfort. Many of the things she would say to me would not qualify as sound advice. Worry, even healthy worry, is not advice. In my mother's case, she was worrying professionally to create health and ease for herself and others. She was also trying to instruct me how to worry in a less destructive way.

Pearl probably should have told me, "Stephen. I'm not a professional consultant, nor a financial planner, sex therapist, marriage counselor, medical expert, or trained theologian. I'm just a simple mother, a Jewish mother, a professional worrier. Don't take my financial advice to heart. Don't get frustrated with my advice. Just hand over your problem and let me worry about it."

All of my brothers and sisters would want to take her advice literally, and follow what she said. Then they would get angry if things didn't work out.

At the same time, we would get all upset about her worrying because we thought she might get ill or fall apart. Many times we tried to save her, stop her, condemn her, or at least shut her up.

I now see worrying was her way of dealing with a difficult situation. She was following her career as a professional worrier. We always thought she was a little Jewish mother who worried only for us.

We wanted her undivided attention. We *demanded* her undivided attention. When we saw her venture out to worry about others, we became jealous and felt neglected. Little did we know at the time that we were living in the same house with a world-class worrier.

Now we know: You can't worry professionally if you do not care or love.

While you cannot worry effectively if you do not care, an excess of caring or emotion can destroy healthy worrying. If you feel yourself becoming too angry, too afraid, too emotional, step back. Postpone the worry. Have some Ben and Jerry's ice cream, and take a bubble bath. Go to a movie, eat your favorite candy bar. Do anything to soften things up, take the edge off. Believe it or not, healthy worry is not about being on the edge. Most effective worry comes from a place of comfort. Not necessarily your conventional idea of comfort, but more like being in the eye of a hurricane.

The key to healthy professional worrying is to enjoy it, but never let anyone know that you are enjoying yourself. The real joy of worrying is that deep in your heart, you trust that the worst won't happen.

After all, if you think or worry about enough extreme possibilities, rarely could reality ever be as bad as what your mind can make up. *The joy is knowing that your worry is not truth and that in the end all will be well.*

Believe me, you will be much healthier if you worry while knowing truly in your heart that everything is going to be okay. Ask God or Spirit to help you. When you worry, adrenaline pumps into your body and soothes you. It prepares you for whatever will happen. Prepare yourself for bad news and pray in your heart for good news.

As mentioned earlier, my grandmother Maya was a deep worrier. Pearl is more of a surface worrier. But compared to other Russian women of Maya's generation, she actually knew when to let things go.

What Pearl and Maya both had in common was the process: *Worry, worry, worry, and let it go. And give lots and lots of love.*

Or, as my old friend George Agular said when he was teaching me how to rebuild a truck engine, and I dropped the truck transmission on my chest, "Steve, how many times have I told you? If it gets too heavy, drop it." The same can be said about worry.

Keep it light, even when it is about heavy things.

The key to worry is knowing that in fact you have absolutely no control over the outcome. This is the real contradiction for a true professional worrier. It is the Zen of Worrying. While you worry with all your heart, know deep down inside, you are not in charge.

The Zen of Worrying is:

Worry, worry, worry, worry, let it go.
Worry, worry, worry, worry, let it go.
Worry, worry, worry, worry, let it go.
Worry, worry, worry, worry, and love.

Riding the Horse in the Right Direction

On the path to becoming a professional worrier, I've made progress. Even Pearl would admit it. Maybe.

Here is a story about how professional worrying can save the day. It shows how much I have learned from my mother.

I planned to try to visit my mother and sister in California. This would be the first time I would leave my Arizona ranch in three years. Each time I previously tried to leave, something came up which prevented me from going. This time, conditions looked good. I booked tickets in advance, and reserved a place to stay in the Bay Area. I lined up someone to watch the ranch in the day. Most importantly, my staff person, Daniel, was scheduled to stay over at night to feed the dogs, water the plants, and watch the ranch.

The day before I was to leave for California, my ranch hand was nowhere in sight. I waited out the day, worrying like crazy. No Daniel. My departure was nearing. Still no Daniel.

I faced a clear dilemma. What should I do? Time to leave, and no one to take care of the ranch while I'm gone.

I began to worry at a rate of about three or four worries a minute. In my more amateur days, before I saw the value of professionalism such as my mother's, I would have freaked out and cancelled my trip. My worry would have been self-defeating.

Instead, I took a deep breath and conjured Pearl. Then I did a Pearl. The hour was 11:00 at night. No matter. I started calling friends and acquaintances to tell them what was happening. I asked them if they knew anyone who could ranch-sit.

I spread my worry around Oracle, across Tucson – even into Phoenix. Still no takers, but a lot of "maybes."

My plane was scheduled to take off early the next morning. "What now?" I asked myself. I'd worried with everyone I could think of. I decided to just go to sleep, and see what might happen in the morning.

In other words, I stayed up late. Worry, worry, worry and let it go. Worry and let it go. Worry and let it go. I must have fallen off to sleep because I woke up and it was morning. I showered, ate, got dressed and drove to the airport to catch my flight to Oakland. I still did not have a ranch-sitter or someone to take care of my dogs.

I arrived in the Bay Area, and enjoyed a large family reunion. I had a great time, and didn't even call the ranch to check until the next day. I felt like I was floating in mid air.

It turned out that my worry had stirred things up. Daniel stayed out all night the night before my departure. When he returned the next day after I left, he was greeted by a ranch full of people who had decided to stay at the C.O.D. because I had gotten them so worried!

Each worry call brought a different person to the ranch. *The key is to worry in a way which the situation demands. Worry just enough to enlist a solution, but not enough to be swallowed up by your doubts.*

Worrying Yourself to a State of Grace: Techniques

I. Pick the first worry which comes to mind. Don't wait for the perfect problem.

The technique of worry and the regularity with which it is performed matters more than the actual problem itself.

Remember that worry does not actually solve problems. The solution happens on an entirely different level. Worry helps you pass the time while waiting for an outcome, and releases bodily chemicals which help you cope. It's healthier than over-eating, drinking, drugs or other addictions.

Healthy worry is not an addiction but a consistent practice. People who worry too often, too obsessively, too deeply, or as if they are solving the problems of the world, are more like worry addicts. We do not seek this type of worry.

II. Know when you are stepping into an institutionalized group worry.

I know these days there are all kinds of groups: AA, OA, etc. But my mother never lets her worry get diluted and distracted in an institutional setting.

This can result in a serious loss of focus. Kind of like a worry orgy. You really can't pay attention to one person at a time.

You can still go to groups, but go more for the company, to realize you are not alone.

Remember, do not go into full worry regimen in these kinds of groups.

If you start to worry about each person as they outpour their problems, you can easily go into worry overload, or tilt on the old worry pinball machine. It's just too much.

Wait until you are somewhere alone or with one or two people. Then you can worry as much as you want.

III. If the worry is actually causing pain or discomfort, stop immediately.

Take a break. Hand things over to a proxy worrier. Don't over-worry. This is one of the things that gives worrying a bad name.

Most people worry excessively, more than they can handle, and more than others can as well. They often move into grief and hysteria.

Healthy worry is not hysterical. At first, when hearing about a problem, you may become hysterical and break into tears. Go ahead. Cry, scream, do what you have to do. Then, when you are done, healthy worrying can begin. You cannot worry productively when you are hysterical or overemotional. Caution is the best patch for the novice worrier.

IV. Begin with small problems.

"Are my feet too big, did I say the wrong thing to her, should I be worrying about this?"

Strengthen the worry muscle before you

take on bigger worries.

Telling worry stories is a good way for a novice to begin. It's a little less personal, and less lonely. It's okay to tell a good worry story over and over again, especially if things turn out well.

People love to hear success worry stories. Success worry stories reaffirm: "Sure enough, after all my worrying, everything turned out fine."

V. Remember, never take credit for things turning out well.

Just remind people that in the right amount, with the right technique, worrying can be a healthy and effective thing to do.

If you are a professional worrier, like my mother, you can inspire people with your worry stories. Think of hunters telling of their hunting experiences, or old soldiers telling war stories.

VI. When sharing a worry story, you can trigger someone who is repressed, frozen, unconscious, or in denial into a good, healthy worry.

The person may snap out of their denial and realize, "Hey, I'm not helpless in this situation. I can do something. I can worry."

VII. Know that it's all transient, fleeting, temporary.

How long this *state of Grace* will last is another matter. Perhaps an hour or two. At most a half-day. No good gunslinger, like the Lone Ranger, ever stuck around too long. There were other towns to save, other crimes to solve, other work to do. Likewise, Pearl Malkin gets on her worry horse, rides from that state of grace, keeping it in her heart, and looks for the next thing to worry about, the next place to share and spread her worry.

"Who was that mascara-ed woman?"

She was the Lone Worrier. *Oy Gevalt,* Hi-yo Silver, and away she goes. And zei gesund.

VIII. Grace, which by the way, was Pearl's mother's name, is not the place for professional worriers to stay too long.
It's not good for the worry business. Besides, it's hard to function everyday in a conscious state of grace. *Remember, wherever there is worry, there is grace. And wherever there's grace, there are angels.*

Angels Among Us

When you listen to an eighty-two-year-old worrier like Pearl Malkin, you might at first think that she should just stay in bed. You might think she should stop taking risks, stop going out on a limb, stop bothering with other people. But then what would there be to worry about?

A life without worry is a life not fully lived.

As I look back to our past, I realize that my mother worried herself and my family's way through many crises. I realize that we are, in a way, blessed, and that Pearl is, in her own way, a kind of angel. Let's just say she has *connections.*

Her connections seem to show up whenever we pass through a worry crisis, and lead us into a state of grace.

As I'm now working on this book, I'm sitting in a café on Coast Highway One in Tomales, California, furiously writing away. I look up and see a sign: *Your guardian angel helps you find a place when you feel there's no place to go. We're always on call for a friend. Angels are with you every step of the way and help you soar with grace.*

I look at the menu; the name of the café is *The Angel's Café.* It's *beshert,* meant to be.

I feel my mother is with me. So are our angels.

I am away from the Arizona summer heat, and my ranch is being taken care of. That's progress!

Maybe we all are angels. All we have to do is spread our wings and fly. Oh yes, and worry a little bit each day.

Eye of the Storm

When I lived in Galveston, Texas, a big hurricane was headed towards us. The town rocked with anxiety. Should we go here, should we go there? When should we leave the island, what should we take? When is it coming?

This energy can all be part of the beginning of a healthy worry process, if it helps calm you down. Despite hysterical weather reports and news shows which resembled twister disaster movies, and after detailed plans to leave, and my mother's numerous phone calls to get off the island, I ended up not going anywhere at all. I found a quiet spot on the island, in the eye of the hurricane, not moving much at all. I stayed put and weathered the storm. We even had hurricane parties where everyone gathered and worried together until the storm passed.

The eye of the storm is a place one comes to when all the worry is done. It is the moment you know that you have done all that you possibly can. Now things are truly out of your hands. The eye of the storm is about something else, somewhere else. After days of storm and healthy worrying, phone calls from loved ones, etc., I could see how the worrying helped dispel the fear and kept me in touch with others, as well as helped me to release needed adrenaline which I would use to board up people's houses. It helped others leave the island, and others to perform the chores required prior to and during the hurricane. Finally, when the storm came in all its fury, after the proper amount of worrying, I would often find myself out on the street, walking through neighborhoods, observing it all, calm as can be, even thrilled to be alive. All that worry helped get me to the place, that very special place, called the eye of the hurricane.

You sit there – still, calm and centered for just a moment, knowing that everything is just as it should be. And for one special moment (don't let my mother hear this), there is truly nothing to worry about at all. I have seen my mother work herself into this state of grace simply through daily worrying. Almost a trance, but in fact, a state of grace. I have actually seen Pearl worry herself into peace and stillness. She was, in fact, for a moment, one with it all. And, if you don't believe it, still and silent.

When the hurricane passes, the worry crisis is over. Put away your baggy dresses and old shoes, go to the beauty parlor, get a new hairdo, put on your make-up and some of your best clothes and step out.

When people saw my mother, they said, *"Look at Pearl. After all she's been through, she still looks great."* After each crisis, Pearl is reborn. Kind of a born-again worrier. Life springs eternal, and doesn't Pearl look great.

In time, the hurricane in Galveston passed, and there was no longer an eye to take solace in. I was now observing the ugly aftermath of the hurricane. Long lines for food and ice, cleanup crews, insurance scams, the whole earthly mess. Now there was plenty to worry about. Plenty to do. I realized that this was what my mother would do every time she made it through a particular worry crisis. She would take a little time to be thankful, get some much needed rest, and call as many people as she had enrolled in the worry process to tell them things turned out okay. Have a little fun with the good news, take a deep breath, and then back to work. There was a whole world waiting out there to worry with.

And Another Thing...

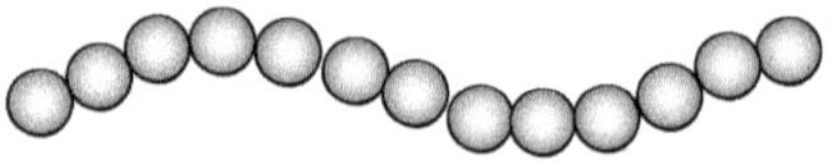

My family has been truly blessed by Pearl's worrying.

Irving got a purple heart, and silver and bronze stars. He raised a family of four with Pearl. Pearl and Irving survived a separation and spent twenty-five more years together laughing, arguing and worrying.

Fifteen years after she was given one year to live, my sister Alexis is thriving – spending lots of time with Pearl every day. Alexis is learning the art of worrying with grace.

My brother Marc, thanks to Pearl's worrying, got to the doctor before his melanoma got too deep to be inoperable. Following successful surgery, Marc is working and raising a family in Southern California. He has learned to listen to his mother and her worrying.

My brother Gary? Pearl is still working on him. He is finally leaving the New Age, and beginning to value Pearl's age-old wisdom of worry.

I finally finished writing this book.

Pearl and I snuck in, and painted my sister Alexis' floor, which has been bare for eleven years – the same amount of years she has been cancer free. I think she believed that if the floor were painted, she would die.

Now, we're worried about whether she'll like the color, but somehow, with Pearl in the caper, it'll get handled.

I was sitting with Pearl, reading her the rough draft of this book, and she wouldn't stop butting in as I read. We got to the part that read, "And Pearl is like an angel." I yelled, "Mom, would you please shut up already."

I paused and thought, "Wait a minute. I just told an angel to shut up." I realized that like Jacob, sometimes we must wrestle with the angels. Worrying is like wrestling with an angel.

LBJ survived Pearl's assassination attempt to die of old age.

Pearl survived her shingles to play tennis daily. She wages an ongoing conversation with hopeless romantics from the Personals columns, but she no longer invites them over. The phone's just fine. Here's her answering machine message:

Hello, I'm sorry I'm not in right now but I'd really love to hear from you. Please leave a message after the beep. Love, Pearl.

Meanwhile, she's still looking for a wife for me.

With Pearl worrying about me, it could happen any day.

P.S. Love Pearl

Well, some time has passed since I finished the initial draft of this book. Finally we are just about to have it published so we can share Pearl's worry with the world. However, before it goes to press, Pearl must share her most recent worry challenge. Let's call it: State Enforced Aging and the California Department of Motor Vehicles.

Pearl Tells All

I was continuing to enjoy my life while sharing as much worry as possible when I received a letter from the California Department of Vehicles saying that they had sent a number of notifications saying that since I was over eighty years old, I needed to take a written test in order to keep my driver's license. I am terrible at taking tests and I haven't even thought about driving rules since I was sixteen. In fact there aren't too many rules I know about other than the rules of a professional worrier. Well this new development triggered a full scale worry crisis.

I studied the exam book, called everybody I knew, and started to hang out at the DMV, sharing my situation with most of the employees. Of course I created numerous worry circles at the DMV and made lots of friends behind the counter. Just think about it. When you get old the state will look you up and try to get you off the road. This is something to worry about, folks. One day an employee came up to me and he said, "Pearl, I'm so worried about you that I'm giving you a sample test with all the answers." I never looked at it but I took it, put it in my glove compartment and forgot all about it.

A week later, a police officer stopped me for turning from the wrong lane. He pulled me over and I began to worry. He asked me for my insurance and registration – and my worry increased because my papers were in the glove compartment with the answers to the DMV written test. I thought I couldn't open my glove compartment, he'll see the test and we'll all get it.

I'll just get him to worry with me and tell him a few jokes; maybe flirt a little like in the old days. Well I'll be damned if I didn't learn a new rule. Imagine at my age:

1. Don't tell off color Yiddish jokes to an uptight police officer.

2. If you're going to worry in a tense situation, just worry. Skip the bad jokes.

3. You can worry about something in the glove compartment, but don't let that stop you from doing what you need to do. Open the glove compartment and show the papers.

Anyway, the officer panicked, did not appreciate an eighty-two year old woman flirting with him, and did not get my Yiddish jokes. He probably has not yet discerned the value of his Irish Mother's worrying. Suddenly, he yelled at me and said, "Mrs. Malkin, you are a senile dumb blonde and I am revoking your driver's license because you are showing signs of dementia. You are too old to be driving." Too old! I'd like to get this schmendrick on the tennis court. But this is like taking a tennis player's racquet away. No more driving to the market, no more shopping at Nordstrom's, no more picking up homeless women and doing their hair and make up and dropping them off. Impossible – Out of the question. I began to build a world-class worry circle. My family, friends, people who I had helped over the years and anybody else I met on the street.

I, Pearl Malkin, Jewish mother and Professional Worrier, was about to be confined to quarters like some kind of elderly assisted living shut-in. Absolutely out of the question. My behavior with the policeman was no different than when I was thirty. It's just that at eighty-two, I'm a little less sexy now than I was in those days. Same behavior, different figure.

Well, we all went to court in San Francisco.

Everybody showed up forming a very nice group worry-circle. There were all kinds of people. My son Gary even brought a lawyer or two. They were all trying to get this judge to worry a little.

I thought, Law Enforcement Agencies and the courts have so lost their human qualities, that they can't even worry with an eighty-two year old woman?

Finally, in a rare worry moment, the judge broke down under the worry pressure and said, "Mrs. Malkin, ordinarily there is nothing we can do, but I am so worried about you living like a shut-in that we will grant you the chance to take a written test and a driving exam. If you pass them both, you can go back on the road."

I was not delighted about this but, what the heck, it was a chance. On the way home a lady drove out of a parking lot and crashed right into my car. You guessed it, the impact knocked my jaw out of place again and totaled my car. You can only imagine. I was already beginning to doubt my status as a professional worrier, but of course I was facing one of my toughest challenges.

It is very difficult to worry professionally about your own personal problems.

Now, I had no car, no driver's license. I couldn't even rent a car and I had to wait three months to take the two tests. In addition, my jaw was so out of place I could barely talk on the phone to mount a new worry campaign.

I decided, okay, I'll walk to the tennis courts. I'll wear a wrinkled tennis outfit, mismatched socks, and carry my old banged-up racquet. I'll call the elderly cab company and get them enrolled in the campaign.

Steve Shares:

In the midst of this, I called my mother on the phone very worried about her being all cooped up in her apartment, all alone with nowhere to go and nothing to do. She said, "Stephen, do you remember when I found that man lying in the road and I called an ambulance and followed him to the hospital, to make sure he was alright?"

"Well, he looked up my name and address in the hospital records and showed up at my door today to thank me for worrying about him and maybe even saving his life. He had a full beard. He said he was a retired teacher and a recovering alcoholic. Anyway, he came over on his Harley Motorcycle, took me outside and said 'Mrs. Malkin, I'll give you a ride wherever you want to go.' I didn't even think, I just got on the back of his motorcycle and spent the day riding all over Marin country. It felt like a jail break - I was free again!"

Pearl said she did worry about falling off, but she had a ball and made it home safe. She almost forgot about all her worries, God forbid. I listened on the phone, worried for a few seconds and then let it go. After all, this is

Pearl Malkin I'm worrying about.

The next day, Pearl walked to the tennis court in her worry outfit and while playing doubles with a younger couple and a friend the ball smashed into her jaw.

She fell to the ground and everybody gathered around her, full of worry. Pearl got up and said, "I can't believe it! It's a miracle." The ball had hit her jaw and knocked it back into place. The pain was gone. Now the worrying could *really* begin.

A few days later she went to the DMV to take her tests. After finishing half the written test she asked if she could go to the bathroom. She came out five minutes later after freshening her makeup and brushing her hair, and of course sharing her worry with someone in the bathroom. When she returned, the DMV official told her they had to take her test away, finished or not, because she'd stayed in the bathroom too long. Pearl started to cry and had a breakdown in front of the entire DMV staff. In a minute or two, she stood up, dried her eyes, and rushed off to take her driving exam. To her surprise, she recognized the official testing her.

He had shared with her about his difficult marriage and Pearl had worried him back to his wife and family. Pearl took a nice country drive with him. He thanked her for all her help and told her "Not to worry!" The DMV would mail her out her test results with their decision in a few weeks.

Pearl rushed home and went to bed, knowing that she had only finished half the written test. She worried herself to sleep.

Weeks passed, and of course she told everybody that she couldn't possibly have passed the written test and that Sunday she was not going to have her license back. What was she going to do?

Finally, the next day, she received a letter

from the DMV:

Mrs. Malkin, this is to notify you that you have passed both your written test and your driving exam and that your California Driver's License is herby officially reinstated. I should have known Pearl was born again – she went out and bought a new car, (well, slightly used), got her license, and immediately went shopping at Nordstrom's, drove to her favorite Chinese restaurant after picking up four or five friends, went to the movies, snuck into a second movie, bought some chocolate ice cream with nuts and whipped cream, drove home, got in the bath tub as she eased the treat into her mouth and smiled.

"Well I guess my new friend and fellow worrier at the DMV was worried about me — that I worried I was old and put out to pasture. That my worried and roaming days were over." My new friend at the DMV said, "Don't worry Pearl" and winked his eye. "What an angel."

Well, Pearl is back on the road, a born-again worrier. She is sharing her life with the people she meets each day. She is free to worry whenever and wherever she likes. Maybe for her eighty-third birthday she'll take a drive from her home in San Francisco to the C.O.D. Ranch in Oracle, Arizona where she'll cook breakfast for my guests. More importantly, Pearl has regained (not that she ever really lost it) confidence in herself as a vital, young-at-heart Jewish mother and Professional worrier who has truly worried her way to good health.

Pearl's Farewell

So, goodbye everybody, I send my love. Please write to me at P.O. Box 241, Oracle, AZ 85623 and let me know how the worrying is going - you never know, I might give you a call.

Love,

Pearl

Glossary of Yiddish Terms

Alta Cocker: Older person; big shot

Beshert: Meant to be

Chutzpah: Balls, guts, nerve

Davining: Rapid bowing while praying

Ferklempt: Stuck; constipated; under the weather; out of sorts

Ganif: Thief

Gevalt: Immense, mighty, terrific!

Hock me a chinick: (Americanized version: Hock me to China); bother someone; talk someone's ear off; worry (prattle) someone to death

Kishkas: Guts; as in "Don't worry your kishkas out."

Kinehora: Knock on wood; worry so you shouldn't have to worry; a curse in reverse (a colleague says "Looks like you are getting the promotion." Kinehora! You cover your colleague's mouth, for to utter such a thing is to ensure it will never happen.)

Kvell: Brag; to express pride in a gentle manner, as for your child

Kvetch: Complainer; whiner

Mishpacha: Family

Mensch: Upstanding human being; someone who will make his/her mother proud

Schlemiel: Jerk

Schmaltz: Chicken fat

Shtetl: Small Jewish village in Eastern Europe

Shtick: Routine; a person's specialty (singing is Barbara Streisand's specialty)

Schmendrick: Someone who should know better

Schmattes: Rags

Schtocken: Tough old survivor

Schtokers: Tough old survivors

Zei Gesund: Be in good health

About the Author

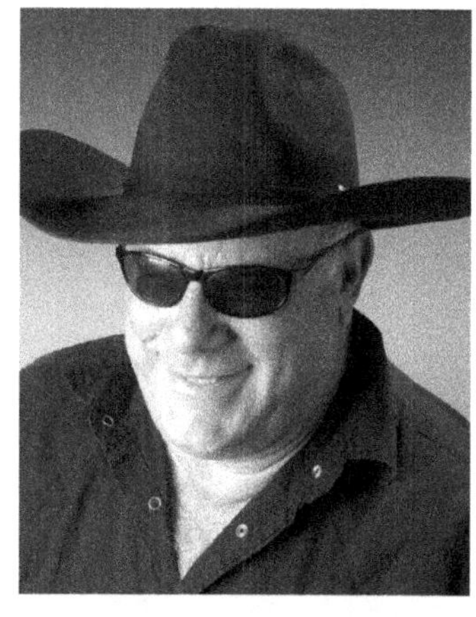

Born in Brooklyn, New York, author Steve Malkin was profoundly affected by his once-orthodox Russian immigrant father's experience living through the Russian revolution. Mr. Malkin is a poet, writer, and master carpenter living and working from his guest ranch in Oracle, Arizona. He has performed his poetry in Leningrad; Paris; Cuernavaca, Mexico; and cities across the American Southwest. His ranch, The C.O.D., plays host to visiting writers and guests looking to use the grounds as a creative retreat. More information on being a guest at his ranch can be found by visiting www.codranch.com.

Worry Notes:

Worry Notes:

Worry Notes:

Worry Notes:

Worry Notes:

www.ingramcontent.com/pod-product-compliance
Lightning Source LLC
Chambersburg PA
CBHW072007040426
42447CB00009B/1522

* 9 7 8 0 9 7 8 7 6 0 8 0 9 *